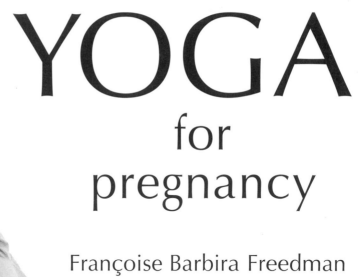

YOGA
for
pregnancy

Françoise Barbira Freedman
and Doriel Hall

WARD LOCK

For the 'wise women' worldwide and our yoga teachers,
in homage to their profound unwritten knowledge.

First published in the UK 1998 by Ward Lock
Wellington House, 125 Strand
LONDON WC2R OBB

A Cassell Imprint

Copyright © Françoise Barbira Freedman and Doriel Hall
Photography © Ward Lock 1998, except for photograph on page 119 © Christina Chelmick
Cassell thank R J Home Stores for the loan of props used in the photographs

Distributed in the United States by
Sterling Publishing Co., Inc.
387 Park Avenue South, New York, NY 10016-8810, USA

A British Library Cataloguing in Publication Data block for this book
may be obtained from the British Library

ISBN 0 7063 7667 6

Edited by Ruth Baldwin
Designed and typeset by Sue Lamble
Illustrations by Roger Courthold
Printed and bound in Great Britain by the Bath Press, Bath

Advice to the reader

If you suffer from any health problems or special conditions,
it is recommended that you consult a doctor before practising any
of the exercises in this book. The publisher and the authors can take
no responsibility for any misadventure resulting from information
given in this book.

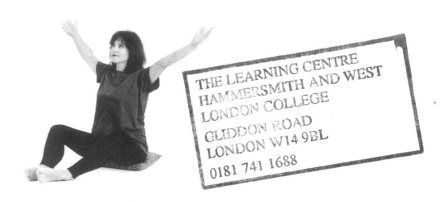

YOGA
for
pregnancy

Contents

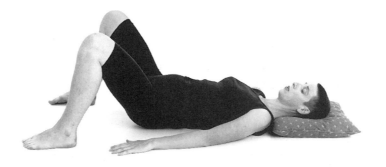

Foreword

Yoga is a science of the inner world of body and mind consciousness. It was developed by the philosophers and meditators of ancient India who investigated that world, shared their experiences with one another and evolved a tradition of practice. Over the centuries yoga enriched all aspects of Indian culture, including the arts, sciences and medicine. Now this is extending to the modern world.

The potential contributions of yoga to healthcare are only just beginning to be appreciated. It can help in the management both of ailments and of natural processes, such as pregnancy. During these nine months many physiological changes occur which profoundly affect a woman's body, emotions and mind. Yoga works at all these levels, helping to maintain physical health and inner harmony throughout this time of intense change and on into the future.

The two authors of this book are ideally suited to write together. Françoise Barbira Freedman has specialized in the application of yoga to pregnancy for many years. As a social anthropologist she brings to it her knowledge of female traditions in indigenous cultures, while as a mother of four children she has direct experience of pregnancy and childbirth. Her yoga derives from a teacher (B.K.S. Iyengar) who emphasized yoga postures and their precise alignment. Specializing for many years in teaching yoga for pregnancy and childbirth, she has utilized this knowledge to adapt yoga postures to the different stages of pregnancy. She has also introduced breathing and body awareness exercises to complement the postures.

Doriel Hall is a well-known yoga teacher in Britain, who has conducted many seminars, workshops and teacher training courses in her own yoga centre and nationwide. She blends precise posture work with the teachings of Swami Satyananda, who emphasized deep relaxation and body awareness. When I introduced her to Françoise (for the purpose of writing this book), it was gratifying to find that she had, independently, come to very similar views to Françoise on appropriate forms of yoga for pregnancy.

While the methods presented in this book were developed through the creative work of the authors, they derive from the basic principles of yoga and are fully in line with mainstream yoga traditions.

The authors' emphasis on breathing practices and body awareness bears out their insight into yoga. Breathing is a bridge between mind and body. Like the heart beat it continues throughout life without a break. However, unlike the heart beat, it can be controlled consciously as well as unconsciously. Breathing patterns sensitively reflect states of mind, and in their turn influence bodily states. By learning to harmonize breathing patterns you can cultivate healthy states of mind and body. Breath control can also contribute in specific ways to childbirth.

Awareness can be said to lie at the heart of yoga. It raises the level of consciousness, integrates the mind and body, and replaces self-centredness by a sense of unity with life.

Dr Robin Munro
Director of the Yoga Biomedical Trust

About this book

This book is in two parts. Part One gives information about being pregnant, and how yoga can help you to get the most from the wonderful process of pregnancy and birth. It is important to read Part One carefully, before moving on to the practical instructions in Part Two, so that you will know exactly what is safe and beneficial to practise at each stage of your pregnancy. All the exercises in this book are chosen to suit the needs of pregnant women – but needs can vary during each stage. Please follow our guidance, even if you think we are being super-cautious! You can get a good work-out simply focusing on breathing.

Part Two describes the yoga practices in detail, with reminders about safety, precautions and benefits.

The Appendix contains explanatory diagrams and a section on troubleshooting. There are also lists of all the exercises in Part Two and useful addresses.

Acknowledgements

Most of the people who have helped with the birthing of this book may not know it. It has its roots in our respective yoga practice, drawn from many teachers. It has been inspired by Amazonian forest shaman midwives and owes a great deal to Corina and Albina in Peru.

Many obstetricians and midwives have given invaluable encouragement and feedback in the adaptation of yoga for pregnancy and birth; although we cannot name them all, warm thanks go to Michel Odent, John Hare, Ina May Gaskin, Roger Lichy, Gowri Motha and Suzanne Adamson. We would like to acknowledge the support of Robin Monro and the Yoga Biomedical Trust in London for allowing the joint creation of this book from live sessions with pregnant women and their partners. Without memorable successive groups of pregnant women and fathers-to-be with Birthlight in Cambridge, the sequences in this book could not have been tested and refined over the years, evolving from shared understanding and the special friendship that birth creates. Rhea Quien, who has been a constant source of inspiration for Birthlight, Regina Guilbride, Bridget Kerle and Margaret Adey as trustees and Sally Lomas and Sharon Honig as co-teachers have offered special support in many ways.

We also wish to thank Helen Denholm for skilfully bringing forth this book as our editor at Cassell while taking part in the London classes during her pregnancy, and our models Alison Gilderdale, Sarah Gillmore, Saskia Kemp and Jeannie Black, who have contributed so much to the individual flavour of this book. Finally our main debt of gratitude goes to the four children we have each borne, whose births and growing up have deepened our respective understanding of 'having babies' and of the intertwined challenges and joys of pregnancy and motherhood.

PART ONE

YOU ARE PREGNANT

This part of the book tells you something about yoga. Many of its techniques have been borrowed by other disciplines – aerobics, 'stretch and relax' classes, stress relief, relaxation and so on – almost always presented in isolation, out of context and without reference to their origin. However, yoga always works best *as* yoga because it is holistic. Its various techniques are designed to enhance each other, combining breath with movement and a positive, relaxed attitude. It is the breath which holds exercise and attitude together, because it works directly with the nervous system whose job is to link mind and body. Achieving this inner harmony of mind and body brings far-reaching beneficial effects during your pregnancy and for the rest of your life. Part One introduces you to yoga and shows you how to organize your yoga sessions.

CHAPTER 1

How yoga can help you

Easier pregnancy and birthing

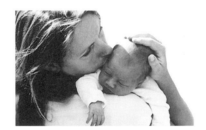

Congratulations on being pregnant! There can be few people – especially first-time parents – who are not overwhelmed by the appearance of a new baby, a new human being created to perfection within the darkness of its mother's womb. So, above all, make sure that you enjoy this wonderful experience of pregnancy and birthing.

Through conception, pregnancy, birth and lactation the body undergoes incredibly complicated processes. All natural processes are nothing short of miraculous, even though we so often take them for granted.

Pregnancy occurs in the body, not in the mind! This fact can be hard to grasp at first, especially if you are accustomed to relying on mental ability and willpower in order to achieve self-imposed goals.

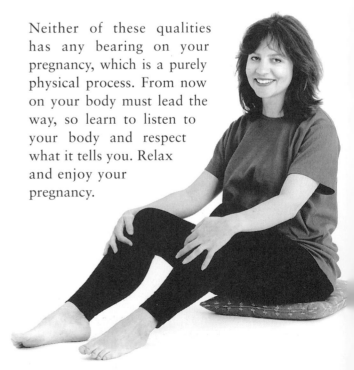

Neither of these qualities has any bearing on your pregnancy, which is a purely physical process. From now on your body must lead the way, so learn to listen to your body and respect what it tells you. Relax and enjoy your pregnancy.

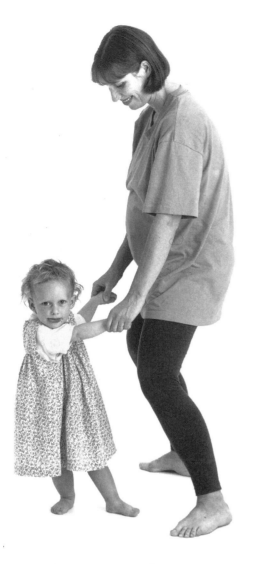

have never done yoga before, you will soon be feeling the benefits.

The techniques in this book were developed for Birthlight. Françoise Barbira Freedman founded this organizaton in 1988 for the 'greater enjoyment of pregnancy, birth and babies', through the practice of yoga during pregnancy. It aims to help women to give birth naturally and joyfully, without undue strain, resistance or fear. It aims to help them to feel fit and strong, and well prepared.

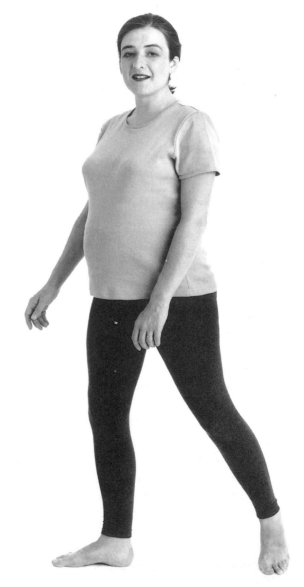

No experience required

Two things are assumed throughout this book: that you have not been pregnant before and that you have not done yoga before. If, however, you are experienced in either of these activities, so much the better.

Every pregnancy is different and so is every teacher's approach to yoga. You will find plenty of useful information in these pages. We have adapted traditional yoga breathing, postures and relaxation techniques to suit every stage of pregnancy, and every level of yoga expertise. Even if you

The benefits of yoga – for you

Among all the methods for easing birth, yoga has the most to offer. This is because yogic breathing connects the action of the voluntary and involuntary muscles in the abdomen. This gives you a control that you could not otherwise obtain. By expanding both your breathing and your stretching capacity, you become familiar in advance with the muscles used in birthing. This will give you confidence, especially if you are a first-time mother.

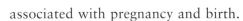

There are other benefits, both in pregnancy and long-term. Your posture during pregnancy is improved and there is a more rapid recovery of good muscle tone after the birth. You will enjoy your baby more because you feel fit and rested. You can expect better gynaecological health in later life because you have learnt how to look after your body during pregnancy.

How yoga works

The main focus is not on the birth itself. It is on *your* health and contentment, as your body undergoes the many natural changes associated with pregnancy and birth.

As the baby grows, yoga is used to strengthen, tone, make space, relax. There is specific training of the muscles involved in the birth. Deep breathing and exercises increase their elasticity and allow these muscles to be pre-stretched. You will learn to recognize, isolate and activate different muscle groups, so that you can use them most effectively during the birth. Different birthing positions are explored, so that you can make full use of gravity and be in control of your own process.

The aim is to achieve a gentle birth through yoga practice. All the parts of the body not involved in birthing are trained to remain relaxed. Control is focused, specific and internal. It results from yielding to, and engaging actively with, the contractions.

The long-lasting elation that accompanies

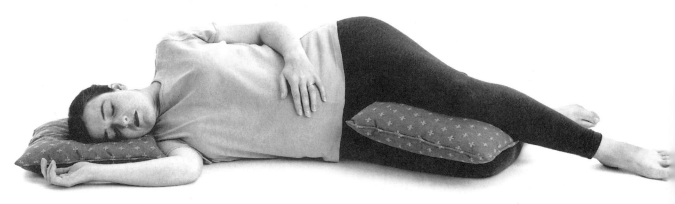

giving birth in this way is extended through you – the mother – to your new baby, your family and your friends. This makes the early parenting phase easy to adjust to. Care during pregnancy contributes so much to your own long-term health and to that of your baby.

Yoga does not stop with the birth; on the contrary! It helps to get your body quickly back into peak condition. It helps to keep you serene and centred, so that you can cope with the problems that a new baby may bring. It helps you to stay relaxed and adaptable, in the face of changing circumstances in your life. It helps you to become more loving and sweet-tempered, for yoga keeps our energies in balance. This results in greater self-confidence and the opening of the heart centre.

The words 'yoga', 'yoke' and 'conjugal' share the same root, suggesting 'united, working in harmony, balanced'. Body and mind are meant to work together as smoothly as yoked oxen pulling their load. The same qualities lie at the core of all successful partnerships between men and women. The yogic state is our own birthright.

The effect of yoga practice continues on into the future and out into the many relationships in our lives. It helps a woman through her pregnancy, the birth and the adjustments to living with her new baby. From there it goes on to assist her in moving back into the wider world of relationships that existed before her baby was born. It helps her to meet the needs and demands of her partner, other family members and, perhaps, her career. An expanding spiral of wellbeing and contentment can result, enabling practical, emotional and mental challenges to be met without undue strain.

Once begun, yoga practice often becomes part of daily life. There are many styles of yoga for you to explore, both classical and modern, with something to suit every temperament and ability.

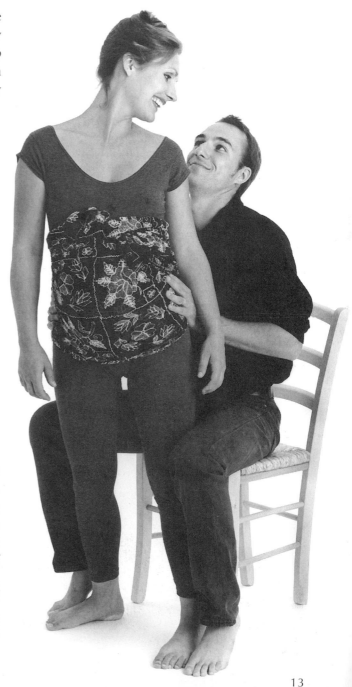

The yogic idea of 'energy'

There are many different yoga 'paths' tailored to balance and enhance different kinds of 'energy'. There is yoga for physical vitality, emotional harmony, mental clarity and so on. These terms describe different aspects of energy flowing through the human system at a subtle level, and from there influencing the physical structures and processes that are the domain of Western science and medicine.

Subtle 'energy' is often called 'life force', because when it is withdrawn from the body life goes too. It enters the body via the breath and also via our food. It is present in light – which is why long, dark winters make us feel low, literally 'depleting our energy'.

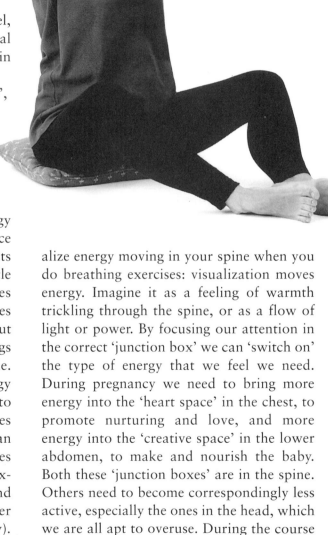

A simple analogy for this invisible energy is electricity. No one can see it: its presence is only known by its effects. These effects can be compared with the effects of subtle energy in our lives. Electricity makes machinery move; our inner energy makes our bodies move. Electricity brings about warmth; our inner energy fuels our feelings and connections with things and people. Electricity focuses light; our inner energy makes it possible for us to use our mind to 'see' and understand. Electricity removes impurities – think of a vacuum cleaner or an ionizing machine. Our inner energy takes care of this need in us through sleep, relaxation, repair of body tissues, digestion and absorption of food (and many other processes that keep us functioning properly).

According to yoga theory, this universal energy has its own circuits in our bodies, with 'junction boxes' in the head and along the spine. This is why you are asked to visu-alize energy moving in your spine when you do breathing exercises: visualization moves energy. Imagine it as a feeling of warmth trickling through the spine, or as a flow of light or power. By focusing our attention in the correct 'junction box' we can 'switch on' the type of energy that we feel we need. During pregnancy we need to bring more energy into the 'heart space' in the chest, to promote nurturing and love, and more energy into the 'creative space' in the lower abdomen, to make and nourish the baby. Both these 'junction boxes' are in the spine. Others need to become correspondingly less active, especially the ones in the head, which we are all apt to overuse. During the course of this book you will be hearing a lot more about 'energy' and what to do with it!

We naturally dissipate some of our energy as we go about daily life. Simple positions, such as bringing the palms of the hands or the soles of the feet together, close our energy circuits so that we can 'recharge'. 'Body language' immediately changes our mood – remember how you feel when rushing to greet someone with open arms, or when you cross your arms and legs in order to 'keep yourself to yourself'?

Breathing and relaxation

Breathing and relaxation are as much a part of yoga practice as the postures, for yoga works on the whole person. Relaxation and stretching alternate, for they are complementary partners. Breath and movement are also complementary partners. This book is full of instructions to 'breathe *in* as you...' and to 'breathe *out* as you...'.

Working in this way increases your own awareness of what is happening within your body. You become far more sensitive to its needs, so that you are able to adjust your yoga practice – and your lifestyle – accordingly. You can thus minimize stress, strain and fatigue throughout your pregnancy.

Yoga breathing for birth develops with practice. Once it has been acquired there is no need for conscious remembering of the techniques. The body itself remembers, at a subconscious level. However inexperienced you feel at first you can – after a few weeks of practice during your pregnancy – look forward to a more effective labour and an easier birth for both you and your baby.

Yoga breathing, stretching and relaxation have a calming effect on the body and the mind. Because yoga integrates body and mind processes, it is also an ideal way to develop healthier patterns of behaviour and thought. Yoga is a discipline that can smooth our path through life in many different ways.

Early pregnancy

First of all – listen to your body. This is a skill that many people, especially in our hectic modern world, have forgotten. As much as possible, it is essential in early pregnancy (also called the first trimester) to live by the rhythms of your own body, rather than by the demands of the clock and other people. Remember that *you* can make this happen. Everyone around you is far more ready to accommodate themselves to the needs of your pregnancy than you may think. It is up to you to admit vulnerability and to seek their co-operation.

It takes about three months for the hormonal changes following conception to take place, and for the pregnancy to be established. The time between the eighth and fourteenth weeks is a delicate

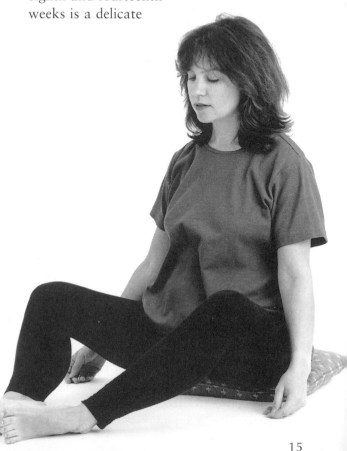

one, when it is particularly important not to overdo it. It is best to avoid all vigorous exercise (even if you already practise yoga). Do the breathing and relaxation techniques (see the suggested session plan on page 26 for what is safe) but drop the physical posture work for the time being. Take walks in the fresh air instead.

You will know when you have moved out of the 'early pregnancy' stage. You will wake up one morning and feel different, that you are now ready to start training for your personal marathon – the birth of your baby.

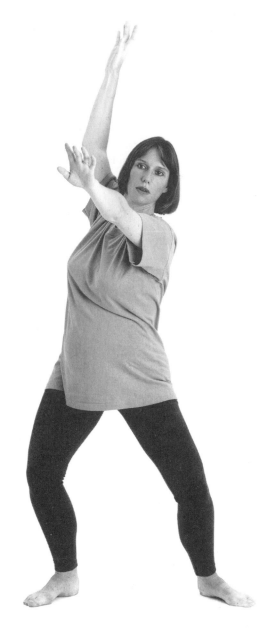

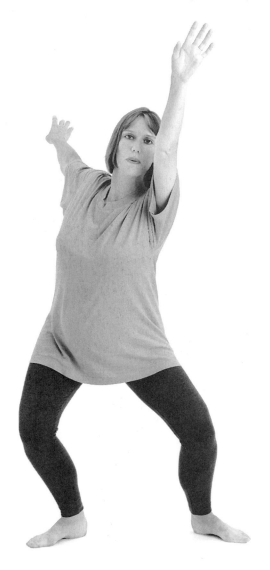

The most important qualities needed during pregnancy are awareness and relaxation, which can both be cultivated via breathing. Breathing rhythms take time to establish, so start early in your pregnancy – even beforehand if possible. Many women have found that the 'letting go' that occurs through working with the breath and practising relaxation actually undoes the tension that may have prevented them from conceiving in the first place.

On the other hand, it is never too late to begin. Even a few weeks of practice during your pregnancy can make an enormous difference to your confidence and sense of wellbeing. Not only pregnancy, but child rearing also, requires that we remain in an attentive and relaxed state, even while doing several things at once. Cultivating these qualities will stand you in good stead through the whole of your life.

Avoiding fatigue and strain

The movements in this type of yoga for pregnancy are unforced and rhythmical. They are usually done on the breath. They can feel like spontaneous expressions of inner joy – yet they are actually carefully designed to build up awareness, stamina and strength in certain muscle groups, while encouraging stretching and relaxation in others.

The focus should be on consciously feeling the body relax into the movement. You should 'encourage' and 'allow' the body to extend, rather than making any effort to 'do'

anything. You will find this yoga quite strenuous at times, yet activity is always balanced with relaxation. This ensures that you feel energized by the end of your session, rather than tired. If this is not the case, you are either trying too hard or forgetting to keep to a rhythm of activity interspersed with moments of rest. Don't forget to breathe! This is the key to awareness and relaxation.

CHAPTER 2

Getting started

When, where and how

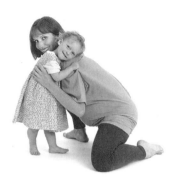

When to practise

Breathing and relaxation can be done almost any time, but you should not practise yoga movements – or any form of vigorous exercise – straight after a meal. This always applies, but you are even more likely to be uncomfortable as your baby grows and occupies more of the space normally taken by your digestive organs. So wait for your food to 'go down'. This will take half an hour for a drink or small snack, and about an hour and a half for a meal. It is therefore best to arrange to do your active yoga sessions before a meal.

Relaxation after a meal is very soothing, as long as your spine is straight and there is no pressure on your abdomen. Gentle deep breathing aids relaxation, but it should not be vigorous just after a meal.

Relaxation in bed is extremely valuable.

You can use a relaxation tape that you have made for yourself to help you to sleep, or simply practise your breathing. A short relaxation on the floor, when you come in after a busy outing, can completely revive you. So can a short deep-breathing session. You can even persuade the family to join in, while you are 'recharging your batteries'.

Where to practise

Always practise yoga exercises on the *floor*. It is almost impossible to sit up straight or to open the hip joints on modern 'comfortable' furniture. The more luxurious it is, the more your chest and abdomen are compressed, your back rounded and your pelvic muscles contracted. Lolling about on such furniture can undo all the good you have been doing by your yoga sessions.

Remember that the purpose of your yoga practice is to:

- Open the chest for deeper breathing.
- Lift the breastbone to make more room for your baby.
- Stretch the legs wide to exercise the pelvic muscles.
- Hold the spine erect for free flow of energy.
- Steady the emotions.
- Centre yourself to cope with change.
- Access the deep relaxation that lies within you.

So make your home on the floor – somewhere warm, draughtfree, uncluttered and non-slip. Take time to find the right place. Is there a cosy corner of your bedroom where you have space to move without bumping into furniture? Or can you reorganize the living room to make your own 'yoga corner' on the floor?

It is a good idea to have everything you need for yoga – cushions, rug, mat or carpet – arranged permanently in your chosen space, so that it is ready for you whenever you have a few minutes to spare for breathing, stretching or relaxation – in addition to your regular daily session. If your floor is draughty or slippery, you will need a special yoga mat or a piece of non-slip carpet to work on – any remnant will do provided it measures about 6ft x 2ft 9in (1.8 x 0.8m). This will also serve to define your space for yoga.

It is best if your yoga corner includes an empty stretch of wall, so that you can sit leaning comfortably against it, put your legs up it, or use it for 'pushing' exercises. Once you get into the habit of settling yourself on the floor for yoga, you can also sit there to watch television, write letters and so on. Every little bit of stretching helps!

Wear clothes that allow for free movement, and nothing on your feet. For breathing and relaxation sessions you can add socks, a jersey or a rug. Avoid jangling

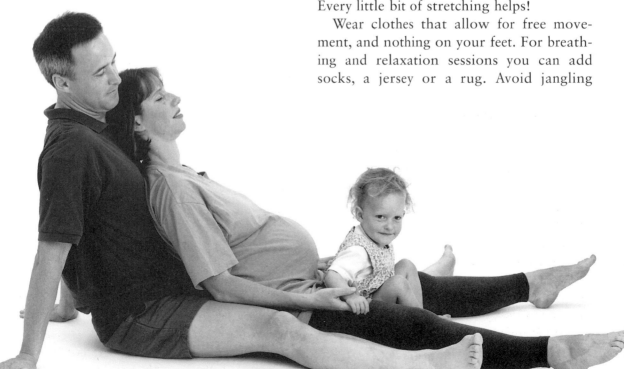

jewellery that may catch in your clothes or constrict your movements. A track suit, or leggings and T-shirt, are ideal. Even if you are not 'properly dressed', you can always kick off your shoes and loosen your clothing for a quick – and probably much needed – breathing or relaxation slot.

What to practise

In early pregnancy – up to about 14 weeks – it is best to err on the side of caution and cut out all exercise routines. It is also wise to cut down on all your activities and take life as gently as you can, resting more than usual. This is the ideal time to learn and practise deep breathing and relaxation in the comfort of your own home – though, of course, you can start on these at *any* time.

After 12–14 weeks, when your energy comes back again, you can start the exercises in this book. They are designed to help women to give birth easily. This training takes time. The more you practise, the better you will come to know your own body and what it needs – and the fitter you will become. Giving birth is a strenuous activity that requires strength and stamina.

Vary your routines, so that the whole body gets a good workout. There are some sequences that will help you to move more easily from lying down to sitting up, to kneeling on all fours, to standing. You may not need these to begin with, but they will be invaluable as your baby grows and you feel more awkward and unbalanced. They are good exercises in themselves, so start doing them even before you really need them.

There are also suitable positions for labour and birthing. The more you practise these, the more they become 'second nature', so that you will go into them auto-matically when the birthing time comes, relying confidently upon the body's wisdom. The same applies to the different breathing techniques: learn and practise them, so that you can benefit from them when the time comes.

Breath and movement should be synchro-nized from the start. The more you relax, the easier it is to work body and breath together – and the more you synchronize them, the more deeply you will relax. Breath, body and mind work together in yoga as interdependent systems.

Integration

You will soon become totally focused on what your body and breath are doing, yet no effort at thinking is required; instead there is a stilling and centring of the mind. This is deeply restful, in sharp contrast to the normal flurry of thoughts clamouring insistently for attention. Thinking takes a lot of energy, so it is no wonder that it can be depleting. Yoga practice gives you time out from thinking, even though the mind is fully engaged all the time – practising awareness of your whole self, and constantly keeping this wholeness in balance.

Pregnancy is a time when hormonal changes, and the prospect of changes in your lifestyle, can cause emotional up-heavals, particularly at the beginning and end. Yoga practice draws all your energies into balance, bringing integration at many levels. It is this coming together of your scattered energies that creates the joyful sensation that so often accompanies yoga.

You get the feeling of emotional integration – a deep and centred steadiness, at rest beneath all turmoil, like an ocean resting peacefully below the waves that scurry across its surface.

You get an even deeper feeling of the integration of experience – whether welcome or unwelcome, all your experiences make up what you are and why you are here. Every pregnancy, however much desired, brings with it some misgivings. These feelings – and many others buried below consciousness – come to the surface in deep relaxation, or in dreams afterwards. They can then be acknowledged with awareness. Deep healing can often take place in this way.

There is an even deeper level of integration – the feeling of being part of life itself, of wonder at the growth of your baby inside your own body, and at the operation of vast cosmic laws and the unfolding of cosmic processes. As you practise breathing into your heart centre during deep relaxation, you become a conscious part of the rhythms of life, of the seasons, of the seas. This is what yoga is all about and why it prepares you so well for the miracle of giving birth.

LIFTING AND CARRYING

For instance, if you have to carry heavy shopping or lift small children, you will know how to use your legs rather than your lower back to take the extra weight. You will become aware of the strength and springiness (or lack of these) in your thigh muscles when you do the routines in Chapter 9: *Standing exercises.* These exercises make it easier to carry the increasing weight of your baby without strain as your pregnancy advances.

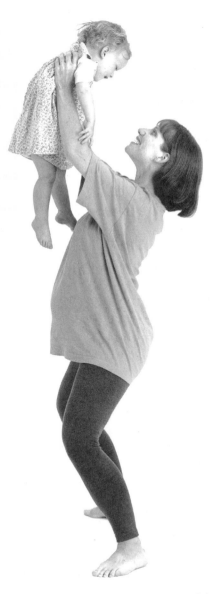

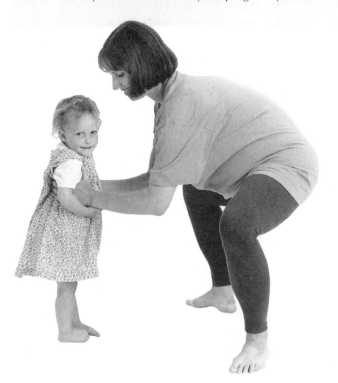

21

Use your yoga any time, anywhere

Once you have learnt awareness of your body, how to co-ordinate breath with energy flow, and how to co-ordinate breath and energy flow with movement, you can practise 'informal' yoga at any time, in any place. You can put your knowledge to good use and develop habits that enhance vitality and wellbeing, rather than deplete them.

Restoring the 'spring in your step'

When you feel tired, remember to pause for a short and effective rest – wherever you happen to be. You will be aware of your own energy patterns and when you have reached the peak of your current wave of activity. It will become second nature to stop whatever you are doing, lift the breastbone to open the chest and draw in renewed energy through good posture and deep breathing.

Remember to stretch the lower back muscles – instead of allowing them to compress – particularly when going up or down the stairs. This strengthens them and makes you feel springy and full of vitality. You will also remember to walk on the whole of your feet, spreading the weight through the soles from heel to toes, with the emphasis on the outsides of the feet. This encourages your arches to rise, which also strengthens the inner leg muscles and the pelvic ligaments. The 'spring in your step' returns as a result of these interactions.

These simple postural habits also help to chase away the 'blues' and to restore your good humour if you become upset or angry.

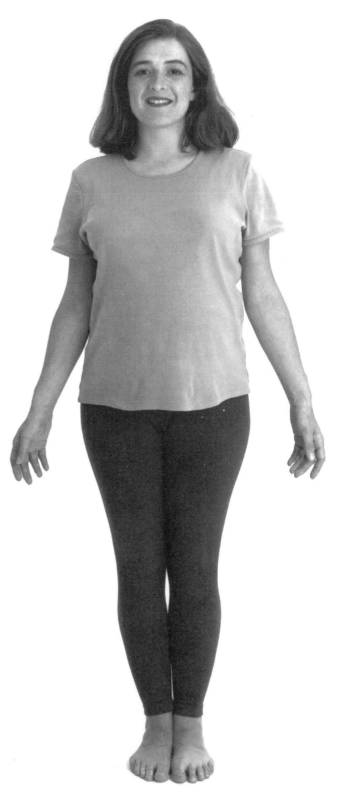

Body awareness

Be aware of the need to stretch whenever some part of your body feels cramped and your energy constricted. You will know how to work that part quickly and effectively, how to loosen up in your shoulders or your hips, how to lengthen and straighten your spine.

You will become more aware of your routine gestures and habitual positions. For instance, you will avoid sitting with one leg crossed over the other, as this cramps the pelvis and squashes your baby. Instead you will automatically sit 'wide and square' with the spine straight. Do notice how you get into a car and have the balance and awareness needed to sit sideways and swing the legs round gracefully, reversing the movements as you get out. This bodily awareness makes you feel centred in yourself and at ease in your own space.

Accepting support when you need it

Of course, you must ensure that you get all the professional help that is available for you and your growing baby, and that you make full use of the expertise and facilities that are on offer.

Beyond this, however, yoga helps you to develop an attitude of mind that allows you to take charge of your own fitness, well-being and contentment. It is unrealistic to leave these things to chance, or to expect other people to perform those miracles that you can do for yourself through regular practice and awareness.

At the same time as becoming more self-motivated and less demanding, you will also become more relaxed – more open, generous and sharing, more ready to ask for help and support when you need it, more 'laid back' as you wait around in clinics or hospitals while the inevitable tests are being carried out.

Yoga breathing and relaxation routines are especially helpful in early pregnancy, between the time of discovery and the time when the pregnancy is well established. A few minutes' practice can steady you, wherever you are. This ability to relax and centre yourself is invaluable during the early stages of pregnancy, when your hormones are adjusting and you are facing many changes in your life.

THE YOGA HABIT

The habit, and the benefits, of yoga are not just for pregnancy. They can last for a lifetime.

CHAPTER 3

Planning your yoga sessions

The right exercises for each pregnancy stage

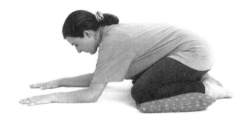

Making time

Aim for an in-depth yoga session every day. The best times are in the early morning, before lunch, in the evening before supper, or before you go to bed. You will find that a few mini-sessions as well are very useful, to rest you and restore your energy as it gets used up. Timing depends so much upon your existing daily routine.

Now that you are pregnant it is more important than ever to prioritize, and to make the best use of your time and energy. You are supporting two lives, your own and that of the baby developing within you. Once it is well on course, pregnancy is a process that we are apt to take for granted. We tend to try to carry on our lives just as we were doing before, but it is advisable to

consider making some lifestyle changes.

Looking after your own health and that of your baby, eating well, resting enough, getting enough fresh air and the right sort of exercise, preparing yourself for the birth – all these important activities must be fitted into your life. It probably means letting go of some of your other activities, even those you enjoy. It may involve feeling 'selfish', as you focus on your own needs, deciding to go out less or to see less of your friends.

It is essential to make space for this baby in your life – and the best time to start is now, while it is being formed inside you; while you are providing the safety of your womb and the flow of your own energies so that it can develop to the point where it can be physically separated from you; while it is totally dependent upon you and is affected by all that you do (or fail to do because you are too 'busy' with inessential activities).

These are hard words – but yoga develops awareness and will help you to discriminate. As you continue to practise you will see for yourself what is important and what is not. Rather than trying to accommodate yourself to the other people in your life – partner, family and friends – ask them to support *you*, so that the making of this baby is a team effort, joyfully undertaken by all of you together.

Planning each session

Besides your main daily yoga session, you will probably also have several short sessions in odd moments. The cumulative effect of all your yoga practice can be truly transformative, greatly improving your overall feeling of wellbeing.

The order in which you do a full yoga session, however short or long it may be, is as follows:

FULL YOGA SESSION

Stage One (Ch 5) *Centring*
Stage Two (Chs 6–7) *Breathing*
Stage Three (Chs 8–12) *Moving with the breath*
Stage Four (Ch 13) *Winding down*
Stage Five (Ch 13) *Deep relaxation*
Stage Six (Ch 13) *Grounding*

These six stages may vary in length from a few minutes each for centring, winding down and grounding, to up to three-quarters of an hour for breathing and exercises and a quarter of an hour for deep relaxation. All the stages should be included in a full yoga session of half an hour or more.

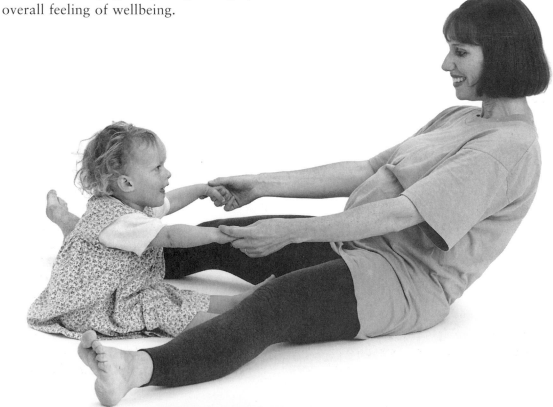

Examples of full yoga sessions

EARLY PREGNANCY (up to 14 weeks)

The following exercises are the only ones recommended for this stage (trimester) of pregnancy:

- Centring (Chapter 5, exercises 1 and 2),
- Learning to relax your body in a variety of resting positions (Chapter 5, exercises 3, 4, 5 and 6),
- Breathing deeply and easily, combining breathing with energy flow (Chapter 5, exercise 8, and Chapter 6, exercise 9),
- Combining breathing with energy flow *and* movement (Chapter 6, exercises 10 and 11),
- Short, deep relaxation (Chapter 13).
- Grounding (Chapter 13).

This may seem an excessively gentle session, but it takes time and practice to get into the 'feel' of yoga. You will be using your time well, and safely, while your pregnancy is becoming firmly established. Meanwhile it is safest to avoid anything vigorous (see Chapter 1, page 15).

MID PREGNANCY (14–30 weeks)

This is your period of greatest choice. Vary your sessions, so that you include all the exercises over a week or so.

- Centring (one or two exercises from Chapter 5).
- Connecting breath with energy and movement (about four exercises from Chapters 6 and 7, or Chapter 8, exercises 27 and 28).

- Changing position (Chapter 8 should become second nature!).
- Get the energy really flowing with a few exercises from Chapter 9; do exercise 30 every time to loosen the muscles around the pelvis.
- Preparing for birthing: do as much as you can from Chapter 10 and a little from Chapter 12. Always include exercises 44, 47 and 51.
- Winding down: include some of Chapter 11, before returning to some deep breathing (Chapter 6) and your deep relaxation position (Chapter 5 or 6).
- Enjoy a long or short, deep relaxation.
- Ground yourself thoroughly.

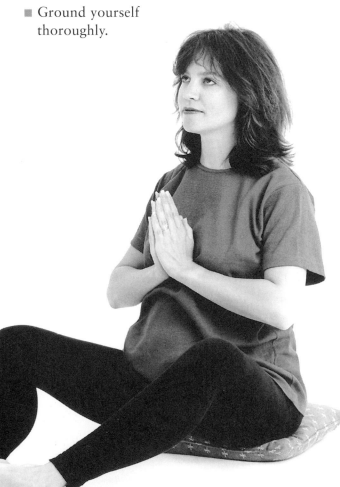

LATE PREGNANCY (30–40 weeks)

You still need to include all the stages, but you may not want to change your position too often. It is important to avoid exercises that involve lying on your back.

■ Start with seated breathing (Chapters 6 and 7).

■ Work through as many exercises as you can *either* from Chapter 9 *or* from Chapter 10, to get a good workout.

■ Work at your birthing techniques in Chapters 11 and 12. Also remember to do your pelvic floor exercises (no. 51).

■ Settle yourself for deep breathing, followed by a long or short, deep relaxation.

■ Ground yourself thoroughly.

Mini yoga sessions

There can be many opportunities for a valuable 'mini session' during the day, lasting from a few moments to half an hour. Get into the habit of making the most of spare moments as they occur. Always practise in the same order, so that it becomes automatic.

Examples of mini yoga sessions

■ Chapter 14 shows a short session which could be fitted into a few spare moments with great benefit.

■ Or you could stand to centre (exercises 27 and 28), and follow with some of the exercises in Chapter 9, sitting or lying down afterwards to wind down and rest.

■ Or you could do the whole mini session from Chapter 10.

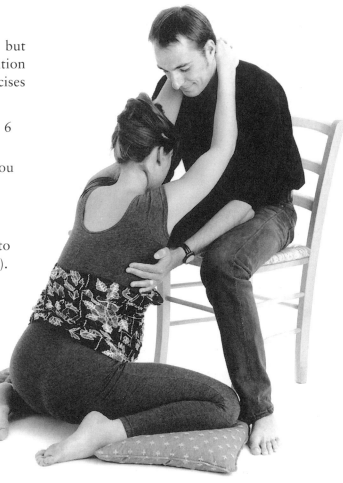

MINI YOGA SESSION

1 Centring
2 Breathing
3 Exercise
4 Winding down

■ Or you could concentrate on birthing positions (Chapter 12) and breath with sound (Chapter 11), relaxing in a seated position for a few moments at the end.

If you have only a short time to practise, it makes sense to stay in the same base position throughout. Precise instructions are given in Chapter 8 on how to change position – from sitting to standing or kneeling and back again – with the minimum of effort. You may not need such advice at the beginning of pregnancy but you will certainly be glad of it during the later stages, when your centre of gravity has shifted. Vary your base position in the mini sessions, so that all your muscles get worked over a period of time.

Mini relaxation sessions

Mini relaxation sessions alleviate tiredness and increase vitality. They are extremely rewarding. The sequence here is:

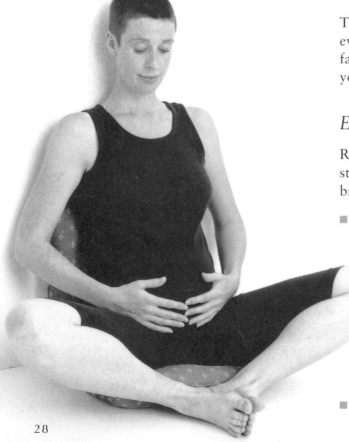

MINI RELAXATION SESSION

1 Centring
2 Breathing
3 Deep relaxation
4 Grounding

The above sequence can be used at any time, even when you are in bed. It can help you to fall sleep quickly, or to get back to sleep if your night is disturbed.

Examples of mini relaxation sessions

Relaxation is always helped by some stretching beforehand, combined with deep breathing and the direction of energy.

- Do a few exercises from Chapters 6 and 7.
  - Start gently with exercises 9, 10 and 11.
    - If you feel like it, become more vigorous for about five minutes, using arms and legs.
    - Return to exercise 9 to wind down.
  - Relax in your chosen position for deep relaxation.
- Ground yourself afterwards.

Again, Chapter 14 is a good example – but this time with more emphasis on the relaxation than on the energetic movements.

Practise!

The more you practise the above routines, the more they will become second nature to you. This means that your body will follow them automatically, with the minimum of effort and willpower on your part. When the time for the birth arrives, you are prepared. During your full yoga sessions you have been preparing your muscles for the activity of giving birth, and gaining strength and stamina. Your mini sessions have trained your body to stretch and relax at any time, so that you can rebalance your energies and stay calm and centred, whatever is happening around you.

These yogic skills will also be invaluable after the birth, as you and your partner – and perhaps your other children – adjust to the presence in your lives of a new baby with its own individual needs.

Family yoga practice

One way to prepare the family for the new arrival is to include them in your yoga practice. Actually, such sessions are extra ones. Your personal practice is all about centring yourself within yourself. Therefore you become introverted and other people are an unwelcome distraction at this time.

Practising with the family requires a different attitude, a sharing of something you all enjoy, preparing together for the new baby.

GUIDELINES FOR 'TOGETHERNESS YOGA'

1 Keep it short, especially with small children.
2 Keep it light: a minimum of explanations.
3 Keep it fun.
4 Keep it spontaneous – no set routine.
5 Do it often to hold their interest.
6 Thank them for helping you.

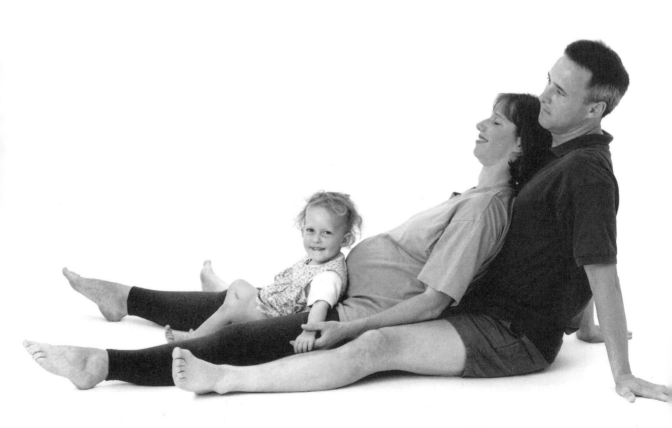

CHAPTER 4

Anatomy of a yoga session

The six stages

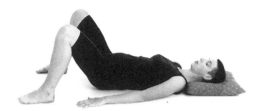

Before you start

Before you start a yoga session make sure that you will not be disturbed. Silence the telephone or switch on the answering machine. Train the people you live with to respect your privacy and need for quiet. Choose a time when you are least likely to be interrupted unexpectedly. Put a notice on the door so that no one barges in by mistake.

Have your yoga mat, or piece of carpet, laid out and extra warm clothes ready to put on for the final relaxation. Arrange all the cushions, and other items that you may need. Have your relaxation tape ready to switch on.

At first it can be quite a shock to be dis-turbed during your yoga session, especially during deep relaxation. With practice, how-ever, yoga will teach you to remain inward-ly at peace whatever outward disturbances may occur. Meanwhile, it is sensible to take precautions.

With yoga you increase:

- Control through breathing practices.
- Stamina and strength through movement.
- Awareness through learning about your body from the inside.
- Calmness and relaxation through focusing the mind.

Stage one: centring

You may like to lie down on the floor to start your yoga session. As your pregnancy advances, however, you will no longer be comfortable in this position. In fact it is not recommended after 30 weeks. After that time you will always start your session sitting on the floor – perhaps leaning back, supported by your arms, a beanbag or the wall. You can put a cushion underneath you, and another one behind you, to make it easier to sit with the spine erect and straight. It is essential to 'sit tall' – in comfort – and to avoid sitting in a slouched and constricted position even when you are not practising yoga.

Yoga always works from the inside out. You are learning to amplify your own inner awareness, and to respond to it, rather than only reacting to stimuli from outside. So the first stage is all about getting in touch with how you are feeling *now*.

Listen to your own body. This may be a new experience for you: as women, many of us have been programmed to consider everyone else before ourselves, and always to put our own needs last. This can make us less aware than we would be naturally, more switched off from our true feelings, yet more anxious and protective of ourselves in unacknowledged and unconscious ways.

After centring, and as a focus for deeper awareness, you will be doing breathing exercises. Awareness and breathing rhythms take time to establish, so start as early as possible in your pregnancy – or even before you become pregnant. It takes several weeks' practice to learn the different breathing techniques. It is also more difficult to learn them once the pressure from the growing baby interferes.

Stage two: yoga breathing

Once you have 'collected yourself' and are feeling relaxed and centred, you will start breathing more deeply. Shallow breathing, which is a very common habit in people with poor posture, occurs when the main breathing muscle, the diaphragm, is constricted and cannot do its job properly. As your baby grows the whole abdominal area becomes rather 'crowded', so it is even more important to learn good posture – to create more space for both your own healthy breathing and for your growing baby.

Your baby needs all the oxygen that *you* can breathe *in*, and to be rid of all the carbon dioxide that *you* can breathe *out*. Remember: you are deep breathing for two!

In yoga we connect breath with energy, through developing our awareness of inner 'feelings' and through using the mind to direct the flow of energy through the centre of the spine.

> All your deep breathing exercises will involve visualizing energy flowing *up* the spine when breathing *in*, and *down* the spine when breathing *out*.

As you breathe gently but deeply, and get a natural rhythm going, you will begin to feel a sensation of energy moving. As you focus your mind upon this movement you will find that you can direct it at will. Mind, body (the breathing muscles) and energy begin to move as one.

This body/energy/mind integration is one of the chief aims of yoga. It is deeply relaxing – and also empowering.

Stage three: moving with the breath

After a few moments focusing on deep breathing, it is time to add stretching movements. Most of your yoga session will involve sequences of stretches co-ordinated with the breath.

First you will use just the arms, in a seated position, then more vigorous movements involving standing, squatting and kneeling. You will build up fitness, vitality and the ability to cope. Through yoga you will develop a well-trained body to be able to give birth naturally and easily, with the minimum of discomfort or need for medical intervention, just as you would train your body systematically if you were aiming to run in a marathon.

You will also become more aware of the need to balance activity with rest, 'doing' with 'being', and effort with letting go. This awareness – carried through into how you live your daily life – is one of the great gifts of yoga. The pendulum should never swing too far in either direction.

Certain groups of muscles need special exercises, together with deep breathing, to prepare for giving birth. These exercises can be done after the more general limbering sequences. (Suggestions for planning your yoga sessions are given on page 26.)

Stage four: winding down

The Western idea that it is virtuous to 'keep going until we drop' makes us far less efficient than we could be. Maintaining a balanced rhythm of activity and rest throughout the day increases strength, stamina and general well-being. It is so easy to continue past the peak of our active curve but, through yoga,

we learn to recognize when our peak has been reached, and to stop for a moment to recharge. That moment makes all the difference. It can bring us back to being 'on top of things' once more.

After completing the yoga movements it is time to prepare for deep relaxation. Your body temperature will drop, so put on extra clothes and have a rug handy. You may want to play a tape during relaxation. Get everything prepared now so that you do not have to move again. Make sure that the telephone cannot ring near you and that no one will disturb you. Make yourself comfortable and get yourself settled.

Always allow plenty of time for this transitional stage of winding down: your relaxation will not be as deep if you go into it with your energies still 'charged up'.

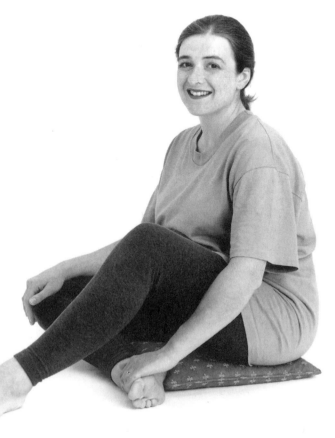

Stage five: deep relaxation

This usually begins with the same deep breathing that you did at the beginning of your yoga session or with some of the exercises with sound in Chapter 11. Your relaxation can take five to 20 minutes, depending on the time you want to spend. It is an integral part of your yoga session, bringing great benefits.

Whatever space of time you allow for your final relaxation, it must be engaged in wholeheartedly. Relaxation cannot be performed successfully with one eye on the clock, or wondering how much time you have left, or when someone will come in.

Stage six: grounding

You will go deep inside yourself in deep relaxation. It is therefore important that you come out of relaxation very slowly, so that you can fuse the deep inner peace that you have experienced with your everyday awareness. Serene alertness is the hallmark of successful yoga practice.

Do be careful to wait several minutes after you open your eyes before leaving your yoga place. You should never rush out and get on with something else at once – you will feel horribly jangled! It is positively dangerous to leap into a car and drive it when you are half-awake.

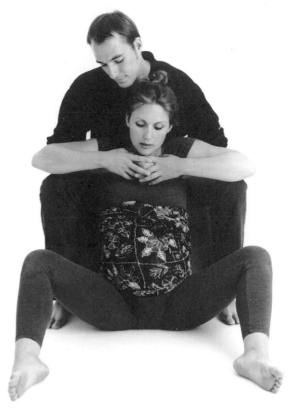

'Togetherness yoga'

These six stages may merge in your sessions of 'togetherness yoga'. Since these are for fun, you will not want to go as deeply into yourself as you would when you practise alone. There will be more emphasis on sharing, and on breath and movement, and less on deep relaxation. The exception is when you and your partner are working jointly to achieve 'togetherness relaxation'. This can be a deep and rewarding experience for both of you.

PART TWO

THE YOGA EXERCISES

This part of the book is practical throughout: yoga is a discipline that has to be *practised* to be effective. You are shown, in simple words and pictures, exactly how to do the techniques, which have been carefully tailored to meet the specific needs of pregnancy. Safety has been given top priority, so that you can work confidently on your own without a teacher to watch over you. Any practice that could possibly be contra-indicated during pregnancy has been omitted, however good it may be for other people at other times. Whenever caution is needed it is spelt out in bold type in a 'Watchpoint' box. Please read through Part Two very thoroughly before starting on any of the exercises.

CHAPTER 5

Centring and breathing

Listening to your body

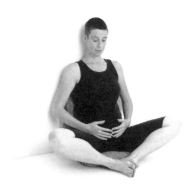

Aligning the body for deep breathing

Once you are centred in yourself, yoga breathing exercises can be used in two ways: to energize or to relax.

The chest is concerned with the breath and the spine with energy flow. Therefore these two areas of the body are always worked upon in yoga. In addition you are pregnant, so your yoga will also work strongly with the lower abdominal area that is housing your developing baby.

The first thing to attend to, therefore, is your posture. Your chest should be free to expand unhindered as you breathe, and your spine should be stretched out and relaxed to allow energy to flow freely through it to your lower abdomen and the base of your body.

Yoga practice starts with centring your attention within yourself, followed by some

sustained deep breathing without movement. The time it takes to settle, centre yourself and relax into your breath will vary, depending upon how you are feeling before you begin. After a few moments you will start to feel energized, ready to move your arms with the breath in Stage Two (see Chapter 6).

HOW TO USE YOGA BREATHING EXERCISES

■ **Do you feel ready for activity?**
Your yoga breathing will empower you to act with less effort and more pleasure.

■ **Do you feel ready for a rest?**
Your yoga breathing will unwind and relax you, so that you can benefit from deeper rest and renewal.

Choosing your position

It is important that you make yourself really comfortable before you start. There are several suitable positions to choose from.

EXERCISE 1

Deep breathing lying on the floor

1 If you are feeling tired, you can lie on the floor. When you are less than 30 weeks pregnant, and lying on your back, you may like to put a cushion under your head (*not* just your neck). This will be more comfortable and give better alignment of the spine. Let your legs lie apart, rolling out loosely from the hips. Your arms can lie alongside your body, resting on the floor; alternatively you can bend your elbows and place your hands on your abdomen to feel the movements of your diaphragm muscle (above your waist) as you breathe.

2 As you breathe *in* your diaphragm contracts *downwards*, making the abdomen swell slightly, and relaxes *upwards* as you breathe *out* (see page 120 for a more detailed explanation).

Since your baby develops in your womb, which is situated in the lower abdomen, you can see how easily the digestive organs get squashed as your baby grows! Much of your yoga breathing and exercise is designed to make more room in the abdomen, through more efficient breathing and posture. This extra space makes later pregnancy far more comfortable.

WATCHPOINT

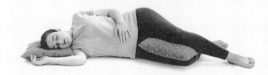

This exercise will be comfortable only up to the 30th week of your pregnancy, which is a watershed. After 30 weeks the weight of the baby can press uncomfortably upon nerves and blood vessels, causing pain or dizziness. From then on you should not lie flat on your back, even in bed. It is better to lie on your side, with a cushion or pillow between your knees.

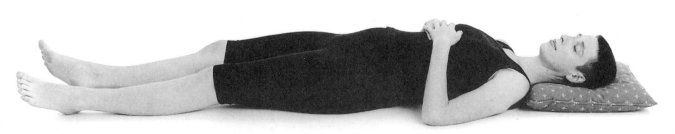

EXERCISE 2

Deep breathing sitting up straight

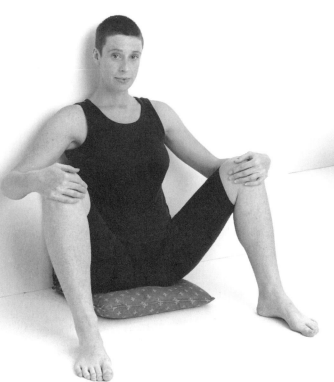

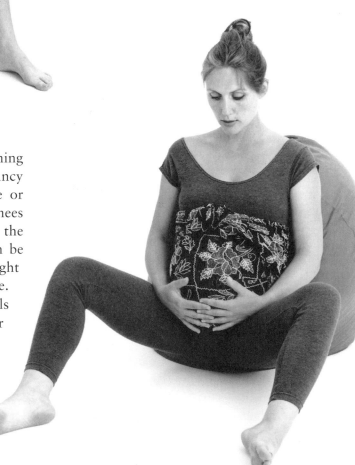

Another good position is to sit leaning against a wall, especially as your pregnancy advances and it is no longer advisable or comfortable to lie on your back. Your knees can be bent up and feet apart, flat on the floor; alternatively your bent knees can be lowered to the sides and your soles brought towards each other – together if possible.

As the baby grows, and your body feels more cumbersome, you can do your breathing exercises leaning against cushions or a beanbag, perhaps with a cushion underneath you or in the small of your back.

Sometimes you may feel more comfortable sitting back-to-front on an upright chair, resting your arms on the chair back. This takes some of the weight off your spine and also opens your chest if you are feeling slumped. (You cannot breathe deeply when your chest sags on to your abdomen, crushing the diaphragm that lies in between.)

The main thing is to be comfortable *and* to keep the chest open and the spine extended.

Experiment with these different positions. Picture your trunk as consisting of the chest cavity, the spine and the abdominal cavity. Your baby is nestling securely against the spine, and is held in place by the abdominal muscles, the pelvis and the perineal muscles at the base of the body. Decide which positions give the best alignment at the stage you are in now. Posture is extremely important at all times, but especially when your body is carrying another body within it.

The position you choose should always allow the chest to open fully and the diaphragm muscle to contract downwards, without constriction, as you breathe *in* slowly and deeply. The diaphragm separates the chest from the abdomen. Above it are the lungs (and heart); below it are the digestive organs (and your baby).

The breastbone (sternum) is like a hinge attached to your collarbones. This hinge should be kept lifted, with your spine

extended, to allow free movement of the breath in the lungs. Your ribs are attached to the sternum in the front and to the spine at the back. In this way they provide a mobile and protective cage for the delicate lungs (see the diagram on page 120). If you sit slumped, this cage restricts your breathing rather than facilitating it.

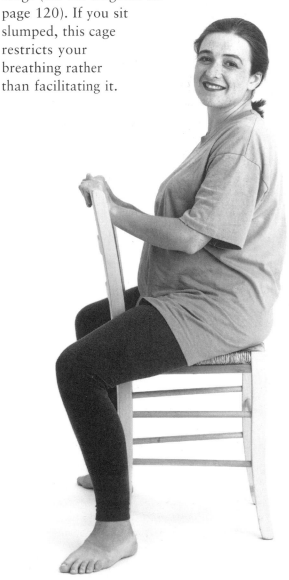

The relationship between breath and energy

In yoga we are also concerned with the movement of energy passing up and down through the spine with the movement of the breath. The processes of pregnancy use a great deal of energy, which should be consciously brought down to where the baby is growing – in the abdomen and pelvis.

Many people, especially if they habitually do a lot of thinking, are apt to concentrate their energy in the head. Pregnancy, however, is an earthy and physical process. Deep breathing brings your energy down to your lower abdomen and the base of your spine, to counteract any imbalances there may be.

Pregnancy is also an affair of the heart: you are opening your heart to welcome this new child that is developing within you. You are gladly offering the safety of your own body and sharing its resources. So you will also be directing energy to your heart centre in some of the exercises and relaxations in these chapters.

Breath in = energy up, breath out = energy down

As you breathe *in*, feel the energy moving *up* through your spine, through the centre line of your being. As you breathe *out*, feel the energy moving *down* to the base of the body.

Here is a very practical way to 'bring the energy downwards' during early and mid pregnancy.

WATCHPOINT

Exercises 1–6 and 8–11 are safe for early pregnancy (up to 14 weeks).

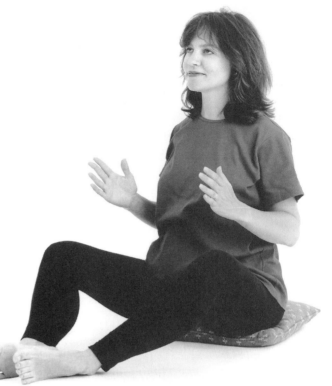

1 Sit in an easy position with hips open and spine erect. Bring your hands above waist level.

2 Now place your palms on your lowest pair of ribs – the 'floating ribs' – with your fingertips towards each other. As you breathe *out*, press your hands inwards and downwards, synchronizing the pressure of your hands with the breath. You will gradually become more aware of the movement of your diaphragm muscle. As it relaxes it lifts upwards into the chest cavity from below. At the same time your energy floats downwards along the spine.

This simple practice is extremely soothing and strengthening. It can bring about deep relaxation in a couple of minutes. Awareness of energy is always subjective but, nevertheless, it is very real – once you begin to recognize the sensation. Meanwhile you can simply imagine it – as a feeling of warmth trickling through the spine, or as a flow of light or power.

Keeping the neck relaxed is very important, because all the nervous impulses that pass between the brain and the rest of the body (except the head) have to pass through the neck. Often we are not even aware that our necks are tense. Remember: if you can go into labour with a relaxed neck, you are half-way there! So it is well worth developing awareness of the neck as early as possible.

Breathe to relax and energize – any time

You should use yoga in your everyday life. There must be many odd moments in your day when you can practise this simplest of routines – sitting with breastbone lifted, chest open and spine extended, so that you can relax and breathe more deeply to 'recharge your batteries'.

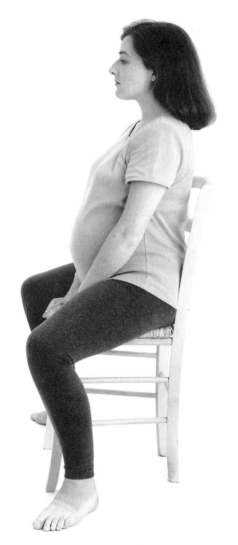

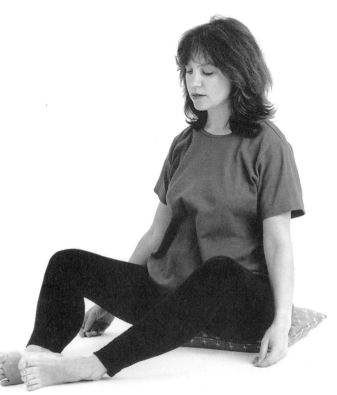

Whenever you are sitting, always be sure to open and spread the base of your body, so that you feel well grounded and secure, in touch with the earth beneath you. When you are sitting on the floor you can open your bent knees outwards, whether you choose to bring your feet together or not. Or you can stretch one or both legs out straight and wide apart, with your toes turned up. It is good to change your position from time to time, while still keeping the hips open.

If you are sitting on a chair, sit 'cowboy fashion' – even if this is not ladylike! Rest your feet flat on the floor and keep your knees wide. Always avoid crossing one leg over the other, as this restricts both blood circulation and the flow of energy downwards. Your hands can be on your knees or in your lap, or curled around your baby.

Focus on breathing *out* to get the energy *down* into the base of the body to nourish your baby. The breath *in* will take care of itself.

Do your yoga gently and without strain. Make use of whatever supports you need to

ensure your comfort, especially strategically placed cushions. As you breathe, let go of tiredness and tension. Let them simply evaporate on the breath *out*, or 'melt away' into the floor as your energy moves *down*.

EXERCISE 3

Upturned beetle

Some people's bodies are so tense that when they do start to let go, through yoga breathing, they can feel quite light-headed. If this happens to you, just *stop* and *flop*! The Upturned Beetle is perfect for this, as the floor is supporting you – but remember not to lie on your back after your 30th week of pregnancy. You will very soon get used to the extra oxygen and energy moving around in your system and wonder how you managed without it!

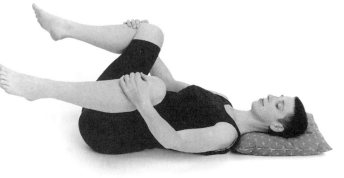

2   Bend your knees and place one hand on each knee. Feel your spine in contact with the floor. Press your tailbone, waist and neck towards the floor.

3   Rotate your knees in small circles with your hands, softening in the hips and lower back.

Brief rest periods are very important for everyone, at any time of day. They allow tension and tiredness to drain away before it can build up. This is a very relaxing position, especially suited to early pregnancy (up to 14 weeks), when rest is the most important consideration. Just lie there and watch the natural flow of your breath, until you feel ready to sit up again.

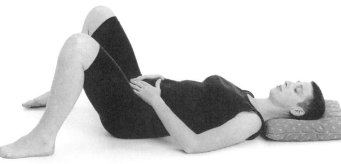

1   Lie on your back with your spine extended and chin tucked in.

EXERCISE 4

Fatigue relief

This exercise is helpful whenever you feel tired, but you should not do it after your 30th week of pregnancy.

1 Lie down on the floor. Place your feet flat on the floor, knees bent. Cross your wrists over your chest, placing your hands on the opposite collarbones.

2 Breathe deeply and feel your upper back opening. Spread it into the floor as you breathe *out*. Release all your tiredness through your back and down into the floor beneath you. After strenuous activity, or in times of stress, you can release your tiredness simply by taking your breath *out* 'down' through your back and into the floor beneath you.

It is helpful to place a cushion or two under your buttocks to soothe the lower back. This creates a better position to allow the breath to expand more, so that energy can flow through the lower abdomen.

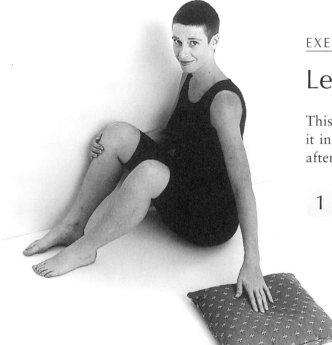

EXERCISE 5

Legs up the wall

This exercise relieves tired legs. Again, since it involves lying on your back, do not do it after the 30th week of your pregnancy.

1 Sit sideways, right next to a wall, with at least one cushion near you.

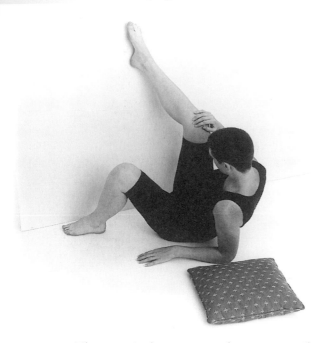

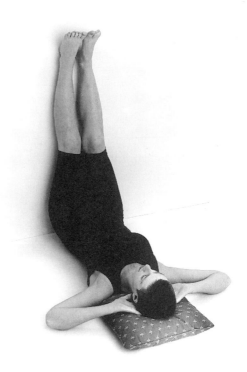

2 Then swivel on your bottom until your legs are up the wall, with no space between your buttocks and the wall.

3 Place your hands under the top of the back of the head (*not* under your neck). This position will open the chest, and encourage you to tuck your chin in and lengthen the back of the neck.

Alternatively you can rest with your legs up the wall and your hands clasped around your baby. If you like, you can gently spread your legs out to the sides. Let them fall as far apart as they will go naturally, without forcing them.

You can place cushions under your hips to invert the body more, and also under your head to release tension in the neck. When you feel 'full of beans', use the yoga breathing exercises to make the most of your energy. When you are tired, use them to unwind and relax.

EXERCISE 6

Soles on the wall

1 Lie on your back (not advised after the 30th week of pregnancy) with

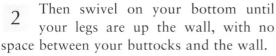

WATCHPOINT

Exercises 1–6 and 8–11 are safe for early pregnancy (up to 14 weeks).

your legs up the wall. Shuffle your buttocks a little away from the wall. Now bend your knees and place your soles flat on the wall. Rest your little fingers on your pubic bone and watch your hands part as you breathe *in* very deeply.

2   Breathe *out* and push your heels away for more stretch. You can focus either on your breathing, by placing your hands on the abdomen, or on stretching in your legs by placing your hands on the inner thighs and stroking them gently to help them to release. They should remain soft as you stroke them. If the inner thigh muscles tense up, it is time to stop.

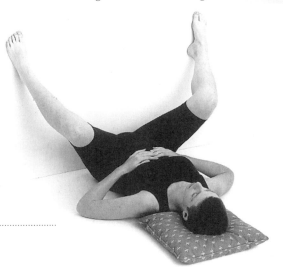

EXERCISE 7

Pushing against a wall

This exercise is *not* recommended in early pregnancy (up to 14 weeks) or after the 30th week.

As your breathing gets deeper and deeper with practice, you can extend exercise 6: Soles on the Wall into an early exercise for 'bearing down'.

1   Lie with your buttocks close to a wall and raised on a cushion or two. Bend your knees and place your soles against the wall. Put your hands on your knees. Breathe *in*.

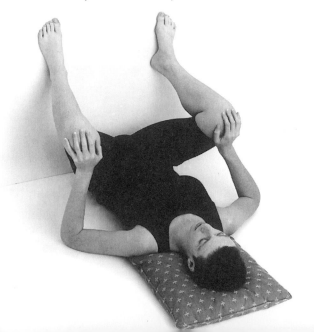

2   Breathe *out* and push with your feet against the wall. You may find that your buttocks lift off the cushion and are drawn closer to the wall. You may feel a small lifting of the tailbone.

This exercise will help you to locate those muscles that you will be using to give birth. It may also help you to understand more precisely how your baby will move downwards from your womb, and through your vagina, into the outside world. Deep breathing in this position allows you to mobilize the muscles of the lower abdomen without tensing or involving other sets of muscles.

When you have finished, change your position. Bring the soles of your feet together, with the sides of your feet against the wall. Allow the knees to open wide. Place your hands around your baby, or on your thighs or your knees. Joining the soles like this creates a circle of energy for you and your baby to enjoy together.

WATCHPOINT

Do not force your knees to the side – your muscles will stretch by themselves.

EXERCISE 8

Closing the circle

You can also create this circle of energy between you and your baby by sitting with the soles joined (or as close together as possible) and your hands clasped around your baby. Relax comfortably in your 'nest' at the end of the day, or at any time when you want to link again with your baby and renew the connection between you. 'Breathe' your baby, drawing energy quietly in and out from the navel. This is a wonderful massage for your baby. You are together in a closed circle of energy and love.

Your partner can help you at this time, by gently stroking your upper thighs in an outwards movement towards the knees. This

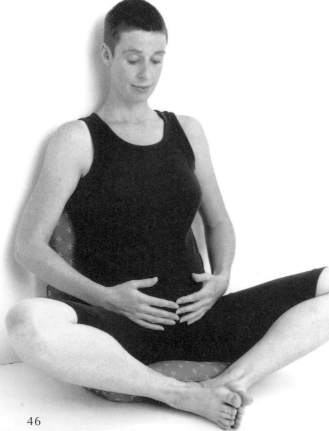

WATCHPOINT

Exercises 1–6 and 8–11 are safe for early pregnancy (up to 14 weeks).

releases tension in the lower abdomen. It also helps the pelvic ligaments to stretch – especially between weeks 20 and 27 – and creates more space around the baby.

A 'work-in'

Whether you decide to sit or to lie down, always start your yoga session with Stage One – connecting the energy in your spine to the flow of your breathing. Focus inwards, deep into yourself. This kind of yoga is not a 'work-out', but a 'work-in' – inwards to the centre of the spine where your energy flows. Every time you breathe *out* it flows through the heart centre and down, around your baby, to the base of your body (where birthing will take place). It rises again naturally every time you breathe *in*.

The same breathing exercises are also a very good way to unwind after the vigorous movements you will be doing in Stages Two and Three. You will be using them again in Stage Four, before the deep relaxation in Stage Five.

Yoga breathing gradually brings inner awareness and integration (see Chapter 2, page 20). It can be a meditation in itself, resulting in deep peace and joy. Yoga breathing exercises are suitable for *all* stages of pregnancy. Start as early in your pregnancy as possible, so that you are well trained in plenty of time for the birth.

CHAPTER 6

Breathing with gentle movement

Starting to move

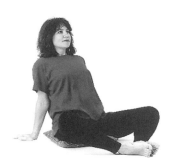

These exercises are to be practised after you have centred yourself in Stage One. They involve breath, energy flow *and* the contraction of muscles, especially in the lower part of the abdomen and the back. You can also use them as part of your winding down in Stage Four, to prepare you for the relaxation in Stage Five.

EXERCISE 9

Seated breathing position

1 You will be raising your arms, so move away from the wall. But continue to use a cushion underneath you, as this lifts the buttocks and makes it easier to keep the chest open and spine straight. If your back feels stiff, sit on two cushions or a beanbag to remove any strain in the lower back. Place your soles on the floor. You can also sit with your knees turned out, which brings the soles of your feet towards each other. Be comfortable! There should be no strain in the hip

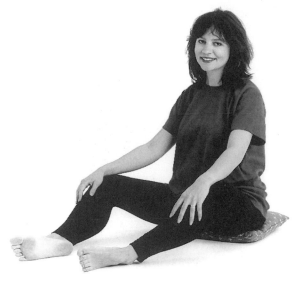

joints or the lower back. If you can, let your soles come together. This closes the 'energy circle', which will revitalize you.

2 Sit with your spine pulled up and chest open. Keep your neck relaxed, with your shoulders loose and down. The longer the spine becomes, the easier it is to breathe *down* into the base of the body and to make contact with it, feeling it press against the floor beneath you. Feel that, as you breathe *out*, you are breathing *down* the spine and into the floor. Practise this for a few breaths.

This exercise introduces you to the principle behind all your yoga exercises: breath, energy and movement are synchronized. The breath *in* causes energy to rise up the spine, the breath *out* causes it to sink down the spine. This will be the pattern from now on, whether or not you are using movements as well.

EXERCISE 10

Breathing hands

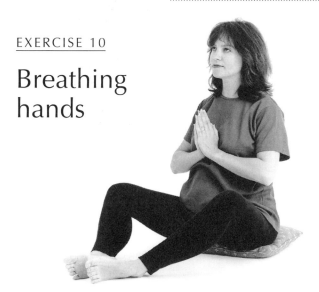

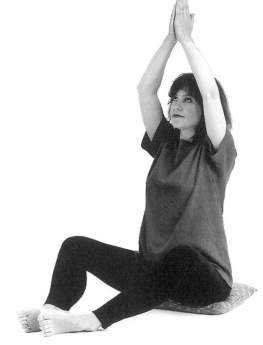

1 Bring your palms together at chest level. Become aware of your hands. Are your rings getting tight? If so, it is time to remove them. The hands often swell during pregnancy, so remember to observe them from time to time.

2 As you breathe *in* take your joined hands above your head. Feel your whole chest open as you stretch *up*.

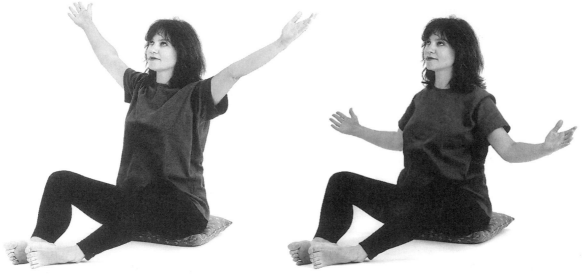

3   As you start to breathe *out*, separate your palms and let your arms and hands float to the sides. Keep the chest open and shoulderblades squeezed together.

4   Bring your hands down beside you at the end of your breath *out*.

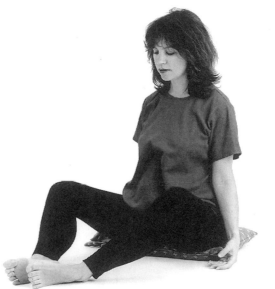

Reverse the pattern, as you breathe *in* again. This time let your hands float *up* to the sides, meeting overhead. As you breathe *out* bring your joined palms *down* in front of you, to rest at heart level.

Then start the whole sequence again and repeat several more times.

EXERCISE 11

The Monitor

When you feel you have gone on long enough, stop the movements. Just breathe naturally *in* and *out* a few times, keeping the hands in front of the heart (see step 1, page 48). Feel that the muscles in your back, along the spine, are involved in each breath *out*. This practice is particularly important if you are expecting twins, as it helps to expand the chest and increase the breathing capacity before the babies start to grow rapidly.

Be aware of your heart beating. Is it calm or speeded up? Be aware of your breathing.

Is it relaxed and deep or tense and shallow?

With practice in awareness you will be able to answer these questions instantly. They are important questions, because your whole yoga practice depends upon knowing the answers. The movement of the breath and the rate of the heartbeats are linked through the nervous system.

If at *any* time your breath feels agitated, *stop* whatever movements you are making and take a short rest, until your breath has slowed down. If you bring your joined hands in front of your chest, you can always check whether your heart is beating in a quiet, even rhythm. You can feel it against your wrists when you keep very still.

When your heartbeat has settled, you can safely proceed.

Use this same check whenever you feel agitated and out of balance, for whatever reason. Just *stop* whatever you are doing and take a few slow breaths to quieten your system down and return to a relaxed state. Yoga awareness allows you to lead an active and physically vigorous life with a relaxed mind and a contented outlook – provided that you act on your awareness and stop to rest when this is indicated by your body.

EXERCISE 12

Chest expansion

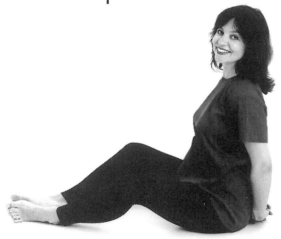
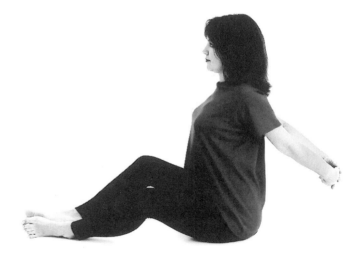

1 Bend your knees and bring the soles of your feet together. Clasp your hands behind you.

2 Breathe *in* and stretch up the spine, lifting the chest. As you breathe *out*, lift your straight arms up behind you, keeping your spine straight.

This exercise is excellent for opening the chest and releasing tight muscles to allow deeper breathing. Breathe naturally, holding the position, until you feel tired. Then bring the arms down and rest, before repeating the exercise once or twice.

EXERCISE 13

Breathing into the heart space

1 Sitting with the soles of your feet together, bring your palms together at heart level.

2 Breathe *in* and press your palms firmly together. Then breathe *out* and press some more. Continue breathing like this, keeping your face relaxed. Be aware only of the sensations in your palms, hands, back muscles and chest muscles. Feel that you are pumping energy into the heart space that these muscles protect and enclose.

After some practice you should be able to feel a softness in the centre of your chest, as you come to the end of your breath *out*. Feel

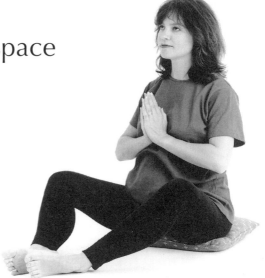

this sensation spread through your breasts. Experience how they are being transformed, enlarging and changing so that they will be ready to nurture your baby.

EXERCISE 14

Breathing into the upper back

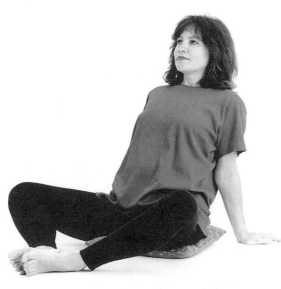

1 Now change your position. Press your hands into the floor behind you, opening the chest and lifting in the upper back. Sit really high and lift at the front. Breathe *in* deeply.

2 Feel that you are breathing *out* in a straight line down your spine. Notice any parts of the spine that seem to resist this flow of energy. Relax into them, bending your elbows and wriggling your shoulder blades and upper body to loosen the spine at those points.

When you are ready, breathe *in* again and repeat the exercise several times more. Your

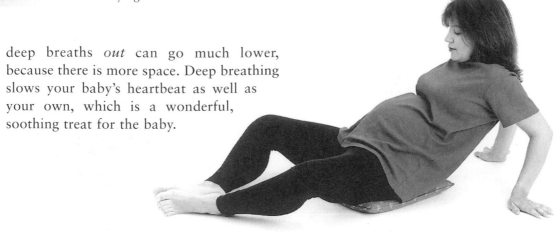

deep breaths *out* can go much lower, because there is more space. Deep breathing slows your baby's heartbeat as well as your own, which is a wonderful, soothing treat for the baby.

EXERCISE 15

Breathing into the base of the body

1 Return to the position in exercise 11: The Monitor (page 49). Sit up very straight with your soles pressed together on the floor in front of you, and your palms pressed together at heart level. Take your attention to the base of the body and bring energy down to this area with every breath *out*.

2 After a few breaths like this, breathe *out* once more and take the energy down into the perineum. Then *keep* it there as you breathe *in* again. Continue breathing and pressing your palms together, focusing on the base of the body. As you increase the pressure in your palms you will feel warmer and heavier in the buttocks, building up a pool of energy in that area.

It is important to learn to 'open the buttocks' and release all tension there, so that you can focus all your energy in the muscles at the front of your body. It is these muscles – not the buttock muscles – which will propel your baby outwards at birth.

3 Return to the position of exercise 14: Breathing into the Upper Back (page 51). Lean back on your hands with your breastbone well lifted. Breathe steadily and deeply in this position for a few minutes. Contract the muscles of the perineum and tighten the muscles around the vagina. You may find that the whole area lifts up. Release and repeat.

These are the muscles that need to stretch to facilitate the birth. When they have been regularly pre-stretched they return to normal more quickly and thoroughly after the birth. Now involve the breath *in*, so that you contract inwards and upwards as you breathe *in*. Breathe *out* as you release these muscles, as slowly as possible.

Remember to relax your neck and lower jaw: this will also relax the perineum, as there are energy links between the lower part of the face and the lower part of the body. Think how we 'hang on grimly' by gritting our teeth! And how readily we relax into a soft smile when we feel safe. It is impossible to relax the perineum muscles with clenched teeth. Since the perineal muscles at the base of the body are connected with the abdominal muscles, you may be surprised to see your whole tummy swing up as you practise this breathing exercise.

EXERCISE 16

Breathing into the sides

1   Next, work to open the sides of the body more. Leaning back on your hands, breathe *in*.

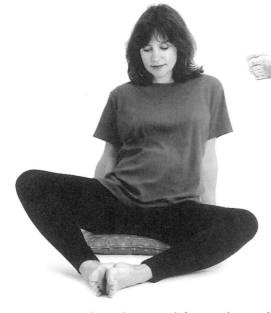

3   Return to centre as you breathe *in*, keeping the spine lifted behind the waist and the chest open.

4   As you breathe *out*, lift the other buttock and experience the contraction one side and the stretch the other.

This gentle rocking movement allows plenty of room for your baby, whilst working the muscles that hold the trunk in place. Repeat the movements several times.

2   As you breathe *out*, lift one buttock off the floor (or cushion). Feel one side contracting and the other side really stretching.

EXERCISE 17

Ankle massage

Gently rubbing the insides of your ankles helps to release the muscles in the pelvis and groin areas.

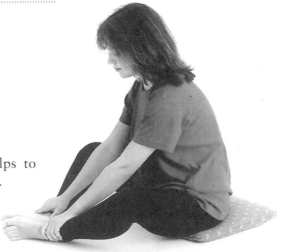

CHAPTER 7

Breathing with vigorous stretching

Loosening the hips

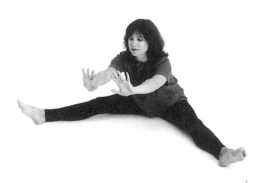

As the exercises in this chapter all have the legs spread wide apart in a seated position, you will probably be more comfortable working without a cushion. Experiment – by moving your legs apart and seeing how far they will go without any feeling of strain. This may not be very far. It is not usual in our Western society to make a habit of spreading our legs wide apart. Therefore our hips soon get stiff and rigid, and the inner thigh muscles shorten so that we are apt to develop 'hip problems' in later life. This condition is rare in countries where people are used to squatting or sitting on the floor instead of using chairs and tables. Looseness in the hips facilitates childbirth.

So start where you feel comfortable. It is amazing how quickly the hip joints will loosen up with regular yoga exercise.

EXERCISE 18

Seated hip stretch

It is especially good to work on the hip joints in a seated position, as the floor takes the weight of the body, leaving the hips free to relax and begin to move more freely. Suppleness in the hips and the ability to stretch the perineum – the 'basket' of muscle that holds the base of the body in place – facilitates the birthing process.

1 Bring your legs as wide apart as you comfortably can, keeping the knees and thighs relaxed. Roll your legs from hips to ankles to iron out any tightness in the thighs that is causing the knees to lift.

2   When you are ready, turn your toes up to stretch the backs of your legs. Clasp your hands together and straighten your spine. Make small circles with your back very straight, like a doll that is weighted at the base so that it cannot topple over. Feel your hip joints loosening. In a few moments you may find that your legs will easily move further apart.

Repeat the exercise.

EXERCISE 19

Breathing into the waist

1   Sit tall, resting on your hands behind you. Bring your legs as wide apart as you find comfortable. Turn your toes up to stretch the backs of the legs, pushing your heels away. Lift your breastbone as high as you can, making more room between your diaphragm and your baby.

2   Breathe deeply into your waist space – or where it used to be! This is a good position to adopt when your digestive organs feel cramped.

When your hips, straight legs, or arms and hands, ask to be released from their position, change it. Sit up, put your cushion under you, bend your knees and shake out your hands gently.

EXERCISE 20

Breathing into the groin

1 Bring your hands in front of you and lift the upper body by pushing into the floor. You can push with your fingertips or, if it is comfortable, by using the whole of your palms.

2 Breathe deeply, breathing *out* into your hands. You can bring them closer to your body, in the crease between your pubic bone and the tops of your legs, so that you make contact with your groin area. Keep your perineum relaxed. You will feel a build-up of energy throughout your whole 'sitting' area as you practise this exercise. After a while you will also become more aware of the various muscles in the groin area.

Your breath *out* is soft – but incredibly powerful. Think of a willow sapling. Nothing could be more yielding, yet it has the strength to break concrete and force its way through.

Allow your own soft breath to open tight muscles in the groin. Breathe *out* to open – then *stay* open. Sometimes, during birth, the baby's head becomes visible, but then it pops back in again because the mother is not using her breath *out* to bear down for long enough. So practise extending the long, strong breath *out* that presses *down*, changing your vagina quite easily and naturally into a birth canal.

Contractions can start with a feeling like a tube train approaching through a tunnel. You will breathe *out* to welcome the train as it comes into the station. Then you will breathe *in* and *out* until the train starts to leave the platform. Then you will breathe *out* 'Goodbye!' as it moves on into the tunnel and rumbles on its way.

These breathing exercises should become completely automatic, so that you can still do them during the excitement of labour itself.

EXERCISE 21

Seated side circles

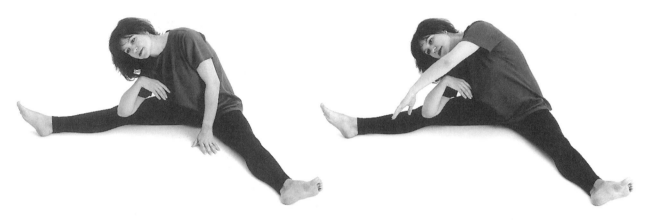

1 Sit tall, with legs wide apart and toes turned up. Place your hands on the floor in front of you. Lean to your right and place your right elbow wherever it feels comfortable on your right leg. (If it won't reach, place your hand on the floor outside your right leg, keeping the elbow loose.)

2 Lift your left arm and, as you breathe *in*, swing it smoothly over to your right side and up over your head.

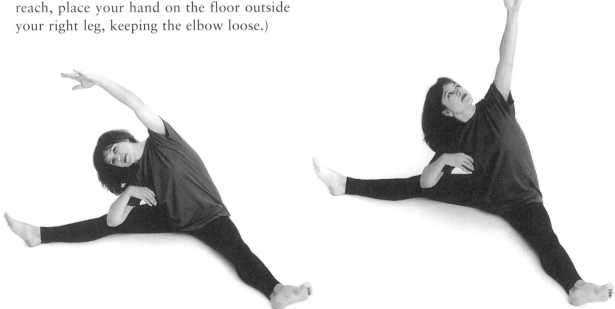

3 Stretch high overhead.

4 Turn your head to look up at your hand.

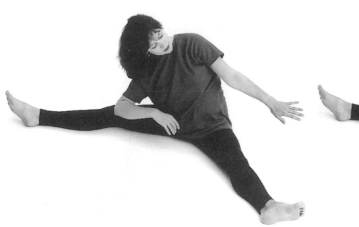

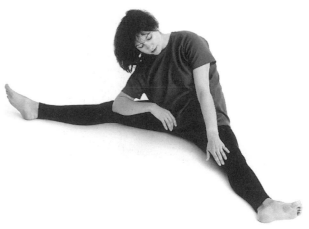

5   As you breathe *out*, bring your arm round to the left and down, ready to start again.

After a few rounds with your left arm, take a short rest. Then stretch up your spine

again, adjust your legs and make circles on the other side. Lean your left arm on your left leg and make circles with your right arm, for the same number of rounds. Then rest quietly.

EXERCISE 22

Seated breast stroke

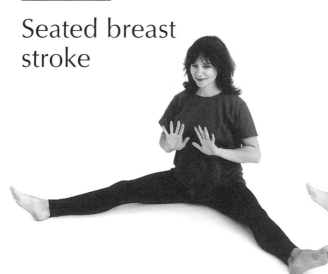

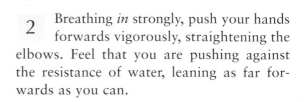

This exercise not only stretches but also strengthens the upper body, while bringing mobility and stretch to the lower back.

1   Sit with feet wide and toes turned up. Bend your elbows and bring the backs of your spread hands in close to your chest.

2   Breathing *in* strongly, push your hands forwards vigorously, straightening the elbows. Feel that you are pushing against the resistance of water, leaning as far forwards as you can.

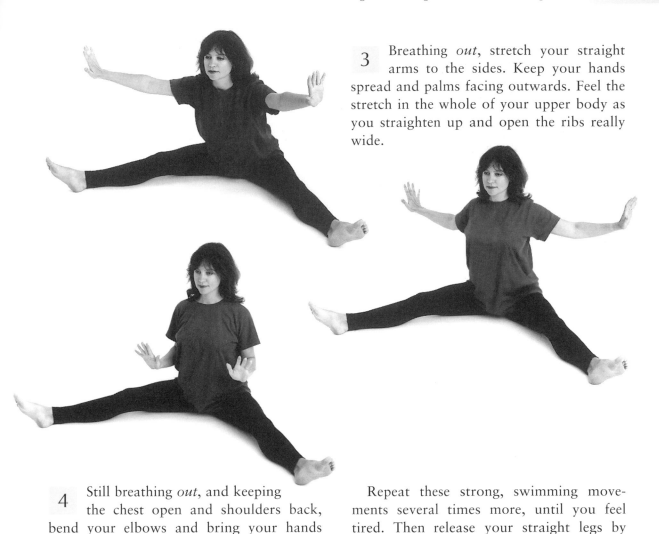

3 Breathing *out*, stretch your straight arms to the sides. Keep your hands spread and palms facing outwards. Feel the stretch in the whole of your upper body as you straighten up and open the ribs really wide.

4 Still breathing *out*, and keeping the chest open and shoulders back, bend your elbows and bring your hands close to your sides, with palms still facing outwards.

Repeat these strong, swimming movements several times more, until you feel tired. Then release your straight legs by bending your knees. Gently (*never* vigorously) shake out your hands.

EXERCISE 23

Stirring the porridge

We are now coming to a more vigorous and exhilarating set of exercises, still with the legs wide apart and the hips open. Exercise 21: Seated Side Circles or exercise 22: Seated Breast Stroke would be suitable 'warm-ups' to do before starting on this one.

1 Sit with legs wide, toes turned up and hands clasped as though you were firmly grasping a huge porridge stick. Breathe *in* deeply.

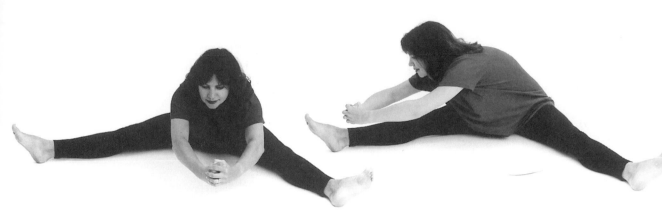

2 As you start to breathe *out*, lean forward from the hips as far as you can go, stretching out your arms in front of you and still firmly clasping your imaginary porridge stick.

3 Still breathing *out*, stir round to the right, bringing your stretched arms over your right leg.

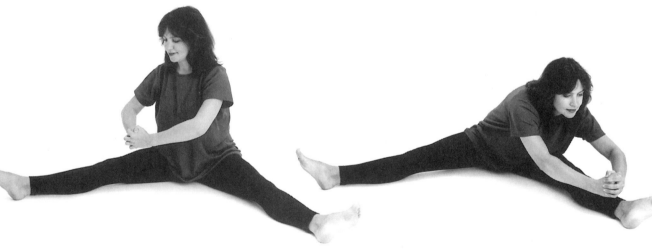

4 Draw your hands back to your waist, breathing *in*.

5 Continue stirring round to the left, starting to breathe *out* again.

6 Reach forward again, still breathing *out*.

Continue round to the right, starting to breathe *in* as your hands come towards your waist. Stir the porridge in the same direction several more times, following this with the same number of rounds in the opposite direction. This exercise should make your breath go deeper and your heart beat faster.

Then rest. Bend your knees and bring your feet towards each other. You may like to lean back on your hands for a moment.

EXERCISE 24

Peekaboo!

In this exercise one leg is folded and the other stretched to the side. This is a comfortable position for sitting on the floor at any time, so it is a good one to practise at odd moments. Change legs frequently. The hips will soon loosen up.

All the emphasis in this exercise is on the upper back, so really stretch the elbows forward and up.

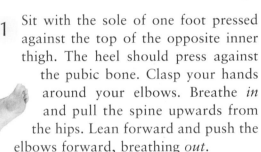

1 Sit with the sole of one foot pressed against the top of the opposite inner thigh. The heel should press against the pubic bone. Clasp your hands around your elbows. Breathe *in* and pull the spine upwards from the hips. Lean forward and push the elbows forward, breathing *out*.

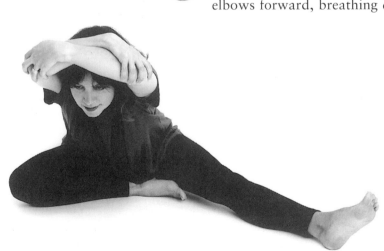

2 Now, starting to breathe *in*, raise your elbows up so that you are looking out from underneath them – until they are stretching up to the ceiling and framing your head.

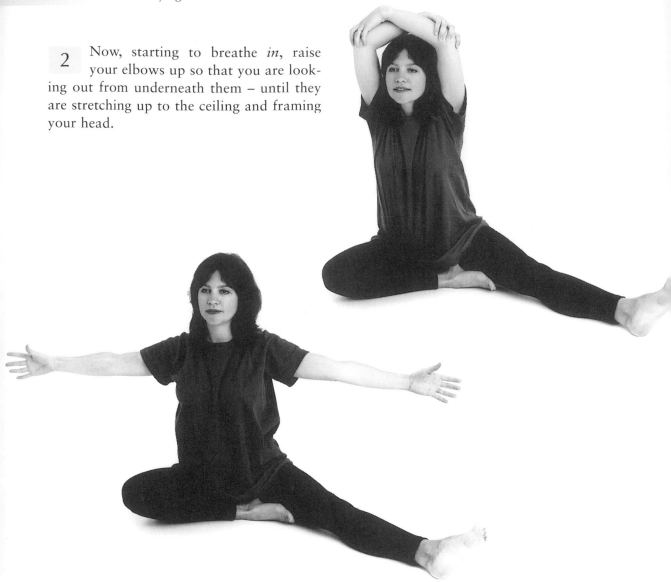

3 Then relax your grip on your elbows and bring your arms down to the sides as you breathe *out* deeply.

Repeat this exercise several times. Then change position, so that your other leg is folded and your other forearm comes in front. This may feel odd – we are such creatures of habit. Then repeat the exercise the same number of times from this position. When you have finished, rest a moment.

CHAPTER 8

Centre of gravity

Changing position

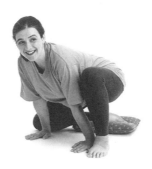

At present you probably get up from lying to sitting, or to standing, with no trouble at all. However, as your pregnancy advances your centre of gravity will shift. Changing your position can become more awkward, especially if you remain in one place for quite a long time. The following exercises make for a smooth transition, and should be practised automatically every time you get up.

EXERCISE 25

Moving from lying through all-fours to sitting

You can use this routine every time you have been relaxing on the floor, or if you sleep on a futon on the floor.

1 Start by lying on your right side. Bend your top (left) knee and bring it to waist level. Bend your top (left) elbow above your left knee.

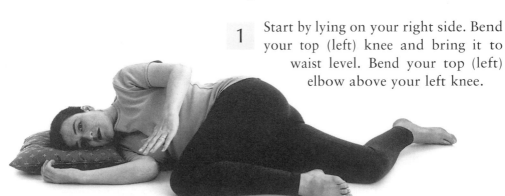

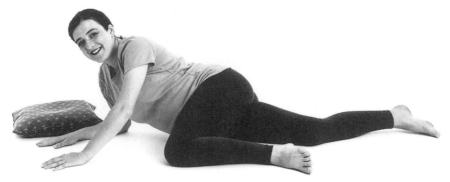

2 Place your left palm on the floor at about shoulder level, and in line with your bent left knee. Shift your weight on to your left hand and knee.

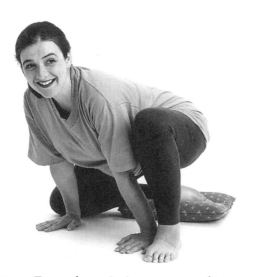

3 As you roll over and take most of your weight on your left knee and hand, bring your right knee underneath your right hip and your right hand underneath your right shoulder. This brings you into an all-fours position – the starting position for many yoga exercises.

4 From here it is easy to adjust your cushion, lean back on to your right heel and bring the sole of your left foot forward on to the floor. This is another excellent way to open the pelvis and relieve stiffness in the lower back. To begin with, this movement may stretch your inner thighs quite a lot more than they are used to.

5 Sit to the right of your back foot and draw it forward to make yourself comfortable in a seated position.

Practise these movements in reverse, and also from lying on your left side rather than on your right side.

Don't forget to pay attention to your breathing. As you go through this sequence you should discover your own natural breathing rhythm, which allows you to move with maximum grace and ease.

EXERCISE 26

Moving from sitting through all-fours to standing

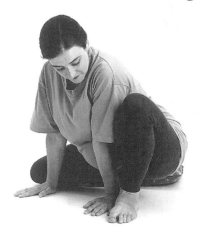

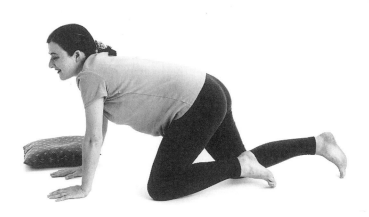

1 From your sitting position with both feet in front of you, slide your right foot in close to your body. Lift your weight on to your hands, and slide your buttocks forward to sit on your right foot. Plant your left sole on the floor in front of you and bring your hands on to the floor in front of you.

2 Take your weight forward into the all-fours position.

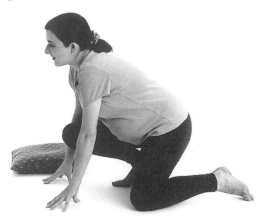

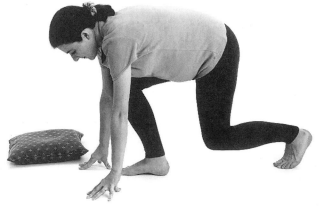

3 Taking most of your weight on your left hand and knee, it is easy to slide the right knee underneath you and place the right foot upon the floor.

4 Take your weight mostly on your right foot, as you tuck your left toes under.

5 Remove all weight from your hands and slowly straighten up to a standing position. Breathe *in* as you stand up and breathe *out* deeply to complete the sequence.

Practise returning to sitting, and going through the whole sequence in reverse. Start by drawing the left foot back and sitting on it.

It is such a pleasure to feel that you are in control of your movements, like a dancer, as your body changes shape, weight and its centre of gravity.

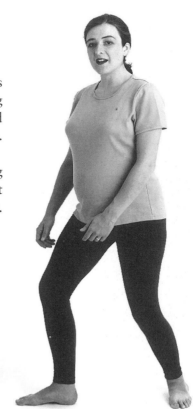

EXERCISE 27

Balanced standing pose

This is one of the classical poses of yoga, which is often done near the start of a session – together with deep breathing – in order to settle and calm the mind. A still mind is more observant, and therefore more aware, than a busy mind cluttered with thoughts. Holding this pose focuses the mind wonderfully, as it is engaged in observing all the minute muscular activity that is required to stand erect yet relaxed, alert yet still. It is a pleasure to hold this pose. It makes you feel strong and centred, well grounded yet reaching upwards.

1 Stand with your feet together and firmly planted. Your big toes should be touching, with your arches lifted and your weight evenly distributed through your toes, around the outsides of your feet and in

your heels. Your feet are the 'roots' from which your body grows upwards towards the light above your head.

2 Slowly draw yourself upwards. As you lift the insteps, the ankles come into line. As you stretch up from your knees, your legs come into line. As you tuck your tailbone under to level your pelvis, your trunk comes into line. Bring the waist back to lessen the contraction that makes a hollow in your back. Lift your breastbone. Drop your shoulders and let your hands hang loosely at your sides. Bring your ears back in line with your shoulders, to lessen the contraction at the back of your neck. Keep your chin level and gaze straight ahead.

Feel that you are being pulled upwards by an invisible string from the crown of your

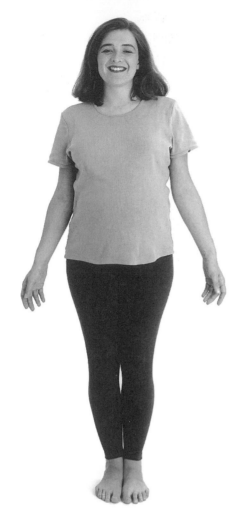

head. Feel that you are growing up out of the ground. The famous image is that of the lotus plant. Its roots are in the muddy darkness at the bottom of the pond. Some invisible force draws the shoot upwards through the water, towards the sunlight. Finally the flower blooms, in all its fragile glory, above the surface of the water. Yet this miracle is being sustained by the roots that feed on the earth beneath the water.

3 This standing pose is a meditation in itself. Breathe calmly *in* and *out*, maintaining the upward lift of your whole body, until you feel tired.

4 Then relax out of the position. Bend your knees and move your shoulders. Rotate your ankles and wrists to ease out any stiffness. 'Wobble' your whole body, like a jelly, shaking it loose while relaxing all over. 'Wobbling' is wonderful for relieving tension during labour.

EXERCISE 28

The tree pose

This pose is a balance, standing on one leg. Have an upright chair handy, in case you need help with balancing.

1 Stand in exercise 27: Balanced Standing Pose for a while first.

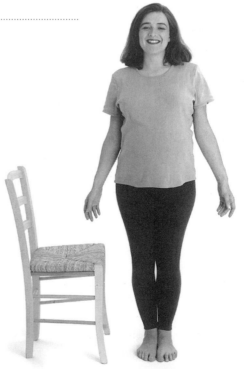

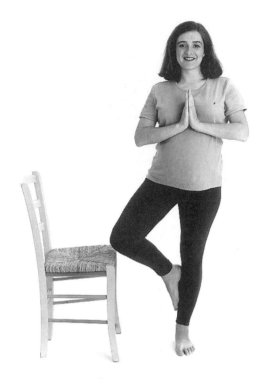
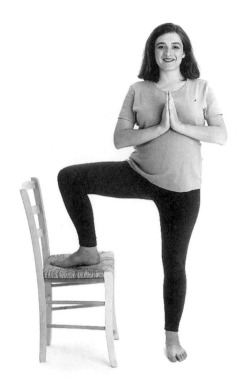

2 Then, when you are ready, draw your right foot slowly up your left calf, turning your right knee out to the side.

Check your balance. If you feel steady, bring your palms together in front of your heart and stay in that position for a while.

If your balance is shaky, use the chair. Place it to your right side and put your right foot on it, so that your knee and your foot point out to the side. Then, when you feel comfortable and steady, bring your palms together in front of your heart.

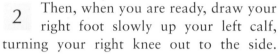
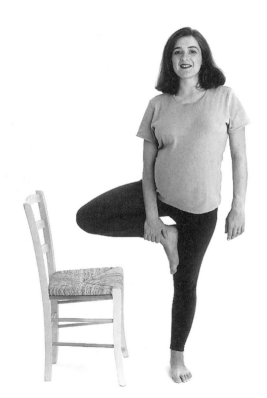

3 You can now come into the classical position. With your right hand, place your right sole against the top of your left inner thigh. Make sure your right knee is pointing to the *side*, or your foot will slip down your thigh. Push your foot against your thigh, to hold it in place.

4   When you feel balanced, raise your arms overhead and bring your palms together. Open your chest as much as you can by bringing the elbows in line with your head, rather than forward, and stretch *up*.

Hold this pose as long as you feel comfortable. Come out of it *before* you start to wobble.

Repeat the whole sequence with the left foot raised and the left knee bent. You may be surprised how different one side of your body feels from the other. One of the benefits of yoga is that it restores balance where we may have unwittingly lost it, through favouring one side, or one part, of the body.

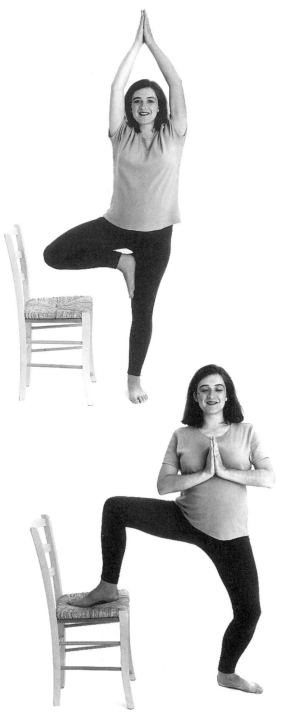

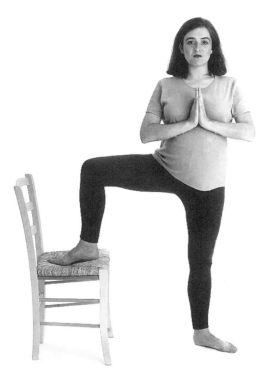

A good variation on The Tree Pose is to take advantage of the chair by placing one foot upon it, as before, with the knee well turned out to the side. Turn the foot of the standing leg outwards a little to protect the knee, then bend the knee of the standing leg.

This is an excellent stretch for the muscles at the base of the body.

When you have finished The Tree Pose on both sides, do some of the swinging, rhythmic sequences described in the next chapter.

CHAPTER 9

Standing exercises

All-over strengthening

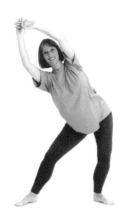

The sequences in this chapter are good for toning, strengthening and relaxing the muscles of the whole body. They give a wonderful feeling of overall vitality and enthusiasm for life.

Include some of these routines every day, from mid-pregnancy on. Do them at odd moments – Charlie Chaplin while vacuuming, Hanging by Your Hands while waiting for the kettle to boil. Vary them, to cover the whole range. Include them in 'family yoga' sessions – children love them. Camel Walking and Hula Hoops brighten the dullest day! Or try Dancing for Joy together in the park. Let yourself go and enjoy the exuberance of these movements.

EXERCISE 29

Standing loose, bending strong

1   Stand erect, but relaxed. Bring your palms together at heart level.

Remind yourself that only the abdominal muscles are needed to give birth, so get into the habit of relaxing all the other muscles. See that your shoulders do not hunch up, but remain relaxed and down – wriggle them around a bit to loosen them.

Your spine should be erect, with tail tucked under, so that the pelvis is level – like

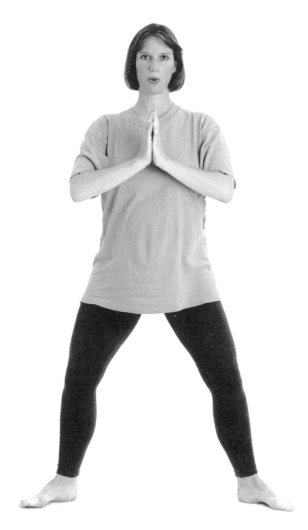

and firmly placed, grounded along an axis that runs from the top of your head down into the floor between your feet. This line of energy passes through the perineum, giving vitality to the spine and pelvis so that they can move freely. You can feel the strength developing along the inner thighs, as the weight of the body is being carried by the legs rather than the lower back.

This is a posture of strength and alertness akin to those of Eastern martial arts, such as t'ai chi. Instead of gathering energy to engage with an opponent, however, your aim is to use your energy to 'open yourself', in preparation for giving birth to your baby. You are in training to be 'strong to yield'.

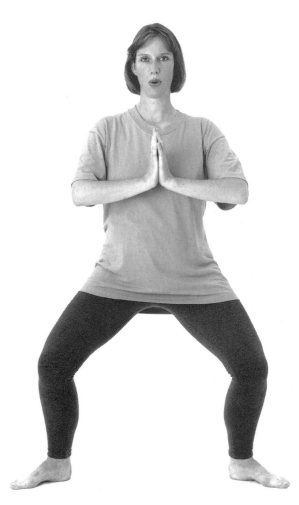

a bowl full of liquid that you do not want to spill. Your knees should be loose and slightly bent and your feet apart. Your toes should be turned out in line with your knees. Keep your weight placed mostly on the outside of your feet and your arches lifted.

2 Practise rising and sinking ever so slightly, by bending your knees and using your thigh muscles. These are the muscles that should support your weight – not your knees or your lower back. So get your thigh muscles active and springy: this is what 'puts a spring in your step'!

As you bend your knees more, breathe out gently. Feel that you are standing strong

EXERCISE 30

The Drops

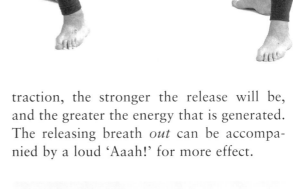

1 Lower your tailbone under and 'sit' on it, as though you had a fisherman's stool or a shooting stick ready placed to support you. Adjust your alignment, and do your corrections, when you are breathing *out*.

At the beginning, it is useful to look in a full-length mirror, so that you can see your side view by slightly turning your head. Your spine should be as straight as possible, with hardly any curve of waist or buttocks. You should be standing vertical, leaning neither forward nor back. Your hands should be loose, with palms up.

Be very aware of your energy – that it is right down at the base of the spine. This grounds you and makes you strong. Keep your knees loose, by rising a little and then lowering yourself down a little more.

2 Once you can drop automatically into the lowered position with good alignment of the spine, add the next – and most important – part of this exercise.

Straighten up and stand strong. Bring your arms in front of you at shoulder level. Clench your fists tightly. Feel the muscles in your arms and upper back contracting strongly as you breathe *in* and then hold your breath *in*. When you need to breathe *out*, release the breath all the way down the whole spine at the same time as you release your body into the lowered Drops position.

The contraction of the upper back and arms is done in order to induce this total release as you breathe *out* into The Drops. The dramatic downflow of energy is what matters. With practice the stronger the con-

traction, the stronger the release will be, and the greater the energy that is generated. The releasing breath *out* can be accompanied by a loud 'Aaah!' for more effect.

TO RECAP

In The Drops, ensure that:

- Your neck is loose.
- Your shoulders are down.
- Your pelvis is level.
- Your tailbone is tucked under.
- Your knees are bent and turned out slightly.
- Your feet are in line under your knees.
- Your arches are lifted.

Imagine a line running straight from your crown to the floor between your feet.

EXERCISE 31

Standing rest

1 *Gently* shake out your ankles and feet, and your wrists and hands.

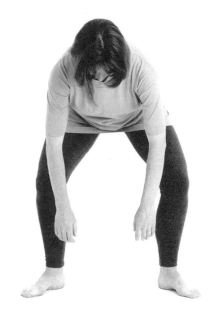

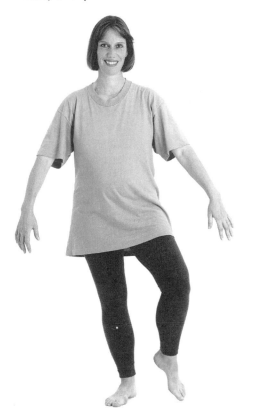

2 You may also like to drop your trunk and arms forward, to ease out your lower spine and the backs of your legs.

All the standing sequences are vigorous, but energizing. Remember: we always have more reserves of energy. We never really reach our limit. We have only to relax again, and more deeply, to tap into our own remarkable depths. By building up strength and stamina we actually make our reserves of energy more readily available to us.

EXERCISE 32

Deep squat routine

1 Bend your knees deeply and lean forward, pushing your 'tail' backwards to stretch the lower spine. Bring your palms together at the heart. Breathe *in*. Think of your spine as horizontal, like a table top, throughout the whole exercise.

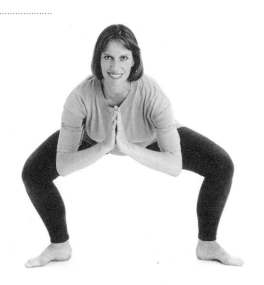

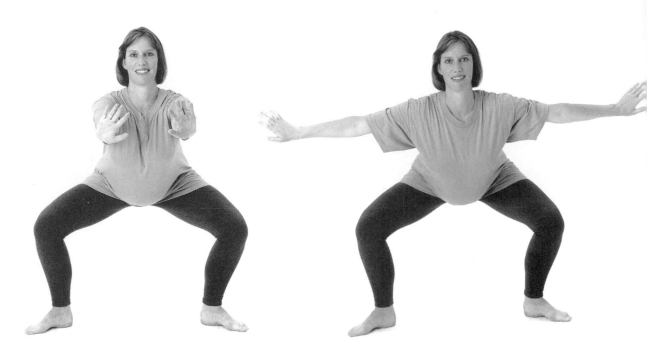

2   As you breathe *out*, straighten your arms and push your palms forwards, as though you were pushing against a wall.

3   Breathe *in* as you sweep your arms to the sides with palms facing out, opening the chest as wide as you can.

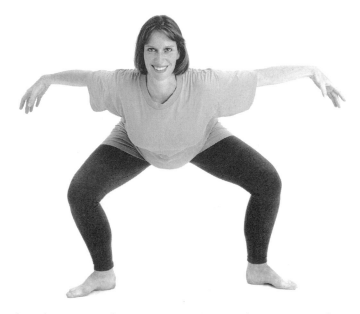

4   Then drop your hands, as you bring your arms as far behind you as possible, squeezing the shoulderblades together to open the chest even more.

5   Breathe *out* to bring your palms together again at chest level.

Repeat these movements several more times, then rest.

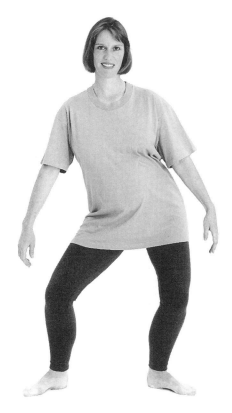

EXERCISE 33

Hula hoops

1 Stand with knees loose and feet turned out a little. Let your arms hang loosely from relaxed shoulders. In this exercise your knees and thighs need to be really springy, so that you can get as much movement as possible in the hips. You will tilt the 'bowl' of the pelvis in all directions – dropping on the right, then at the back (tucking under), then on the left, then in the front (sticking the tailbone out).

2 Swing the pelvis round in circles one way a few times, then change direction and swing the pelvis round the other way.

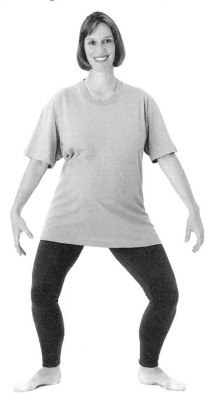

This is a very invigorating movement, which lifts tiredness and is good fun. Children love it!

EXERCISE 34

Lassoing

This is an extension of the preceding exercise.

Be sure to 'lasso' vigorously the same number of times in each direction, or you will feel lop-sided.

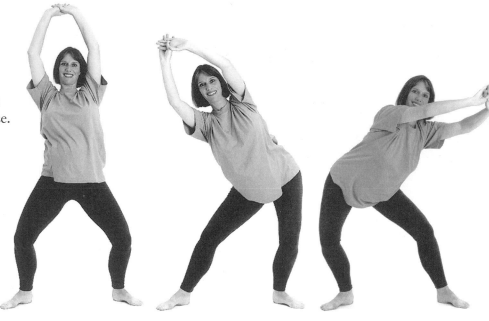

1 Clasp your hands overhead as though you were holding a rope.

2 As you tilt your pelvis one way, swing your arms the other way, keeping your hands together.

EXERCISE 35

Rag doll

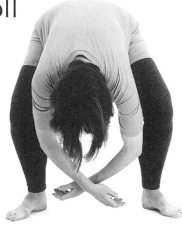

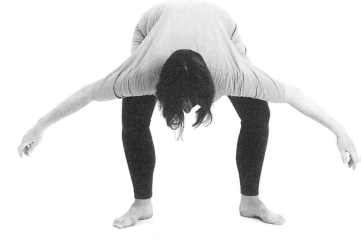

1 With your knees loose and feet apart, hang forward from your hips. Keep your shoulders and neck loose. Keep moving, so that your whole body loosens and relaxes more and more.

2 Swing your arms, crossing them over, then out to the sides, then crossing them the other way. Do several swings, until you feel really relaxed and loosened up.

EXERCISE 36

Charlie Chaplin

In this exercise you walk forward, exaggeratedly dropping the hip of the bent leg. This exercise opens the hips and makes more space for the baby. It can be a great relief during labour, between contractions. It is also very good to do between other standing exercises as it brings your weight into your thighs, relieving your lower back.

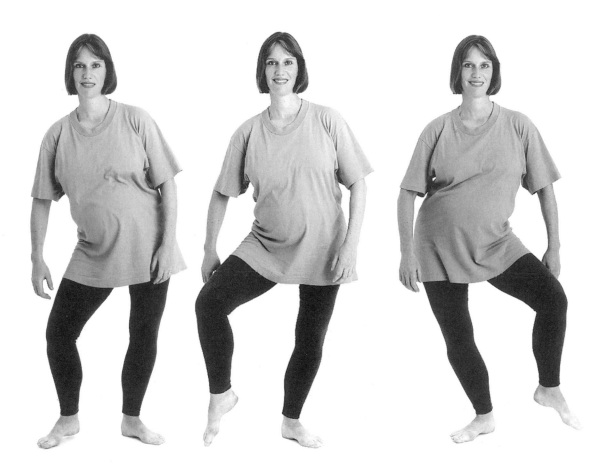

1   Keep your whole body relaxed – especially face, neck, shoulders and arms. Bend your right knee, rotate it out to the right and then step forward, dropping the right hip.

2   Stand on your right foot and raise your left knee. Rotate it out to the left and then step forward on to your left foot.

EXERCISE 37

Dancing for joy

This exercise is similar to the preceding one, but also involves the arms. In it you express joy and wellbeing! It also loosens up the whole body, opening the hips and shoulders especially.

Do these high steps several times, to really strengthen and energize your body.

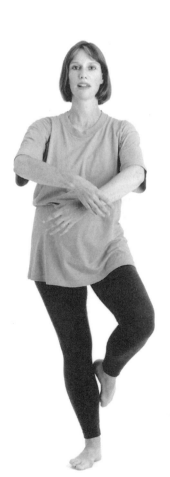

2 As you breathe *in*, raise your left knee as high as you can to the left side and bring your arms up overhead. This opens the chest as well as the hips.

1 Stand with your arms loosely crossed in front of you.

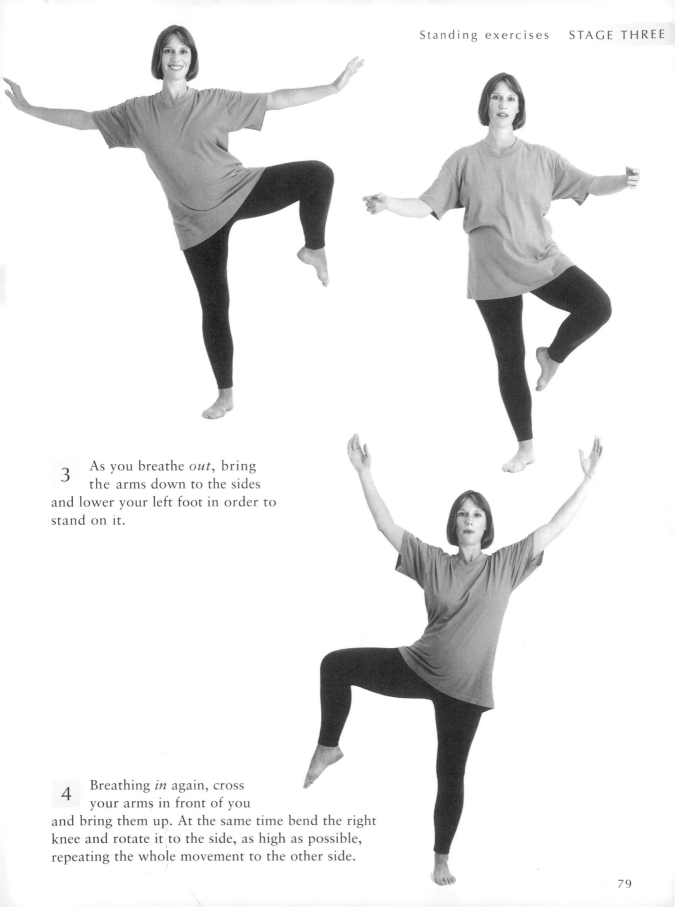

3   As you breathe *out*, bring
      the arms down to the sides
and lower your left foot in order to
stand on it.

4   Breathing *in* again, cross
      your arms in front of you
and bring them up. At the same time bend the right
knee and rotate it to the side, as high as possible,
repeating the whole movement to the other side.

79

EXERCISE 38

Pushing hands

This is a very graceful set of movements that works strongly on the upper back and shoulders, to make more space in the chest and more room for your baby. It also strengthens the vertical muscles in the abdomen, so it is particularly helpful if you are carrying a large baby or twins.

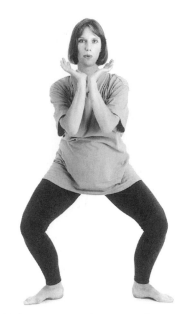

1 Bring your wrists together at shoulder level, under your chin. Turn the palms up and fingers outwards.

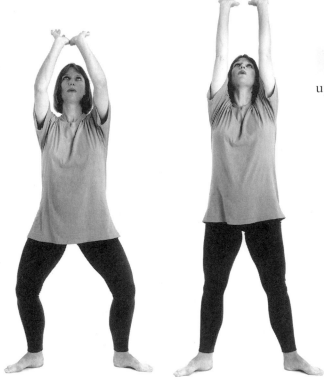

2 Breathe *in* and push your palms towards the ceiling, straightening your legs.

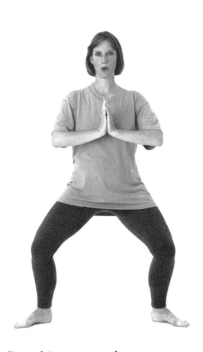

3 Breathing *out*, take your arms to the sides to bring them down, then join your palms in front of your chest and rest a moment, keeping your knees well bent.

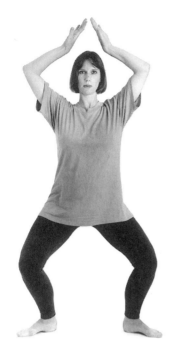

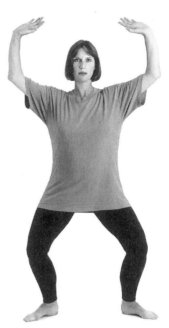

4 Keeping your knees bent, breathe *in* and bring the backs of the hands towards each other above your head. The elbows should be well bent and facing out to the sides.

5 Breathing *out*, stretch the forearms out to the sides at shoulder level, with the palms still facing outwards. You may feel a stretch in your middle fingers as you do this movement.

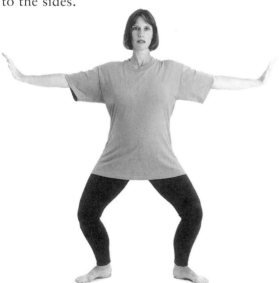

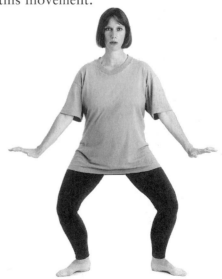

6 Breathe *in* and push your palms strongly out to the sides.

7 Breath *out* as you push your palms downwards, then circle your hands back to the centre with the wrists touching and the palms facing upwards.

Repeat the sequence several times. Each time stretch your arms slightly further down, until your wrists are close to your thighs. Then rest a moment. If you are feeling energetic, but find that standing is too strenuous, this exercise can be done sitting on a stool or chair.

EXERCISE 39

Pulling down the rope

1 Breathe *in* and take your hands up, straightening your legs.

2 As you breathe *out* again, bend your knees and bring your fists down, really *pulling* on an imaginary rope!

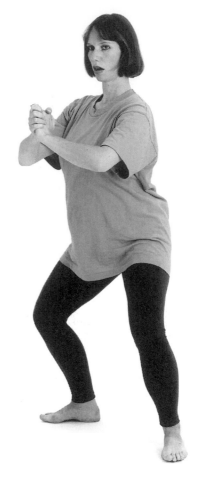

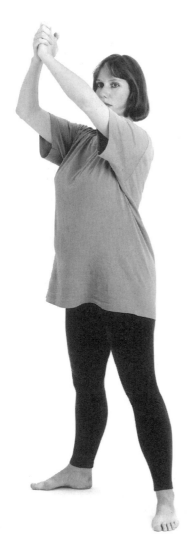

3 Stand very strong and firm, with knees well bent and feet out to the sides. Hold your clasped hands in front of you as if you really were pulling down on that rope. Feel the muscles working behind your heart. Bend your knees and breathe *out* as you go down. As you heart area becomes energized, you begin to feel how you will use gravity to ease your baby's birth.

Repeat this exercise several times, then rest in The Drops (see page 72) with knees and arms loose.

EXERCISE 40

Hanging by your hands

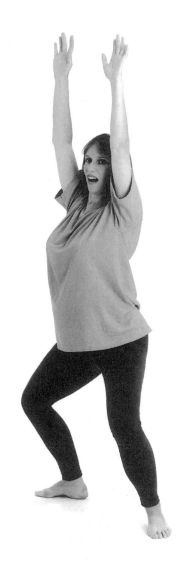

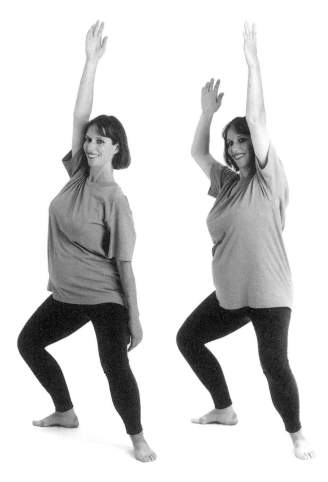

1   With knees well bent in The Drops position, raise your right arm as you breathe in and stretch it up overhead.

2   Then bring it down a little way, breathing *out*, and stretch up your left arm next time you breathe *in*. Imagine that you are climbing a rope ladder, using only your arms. Every time you reach up and grab hold you are extending one side of the ribcage, and relaxing it as you reach up on the other side.

3   After alternating arms for a few breaths, keeping the knees well bent and the hips down, stretch up both arms as you breathe *in*.

4   Breathe deeply into the muscles between your ribs, allowing for greater expansion as the ribs are lifted up and outwards on each breath *in*. As you stretch up, keep the lower part of your body loose and relaxed, as though you were hanging by your hands from a rail.

EXERCISE 41

Camel wobble

Here is another exercise that is very useful for relaxing after doing strong standing poses or between contractions during labour.

In a standing position with knees bent, tip your pelvis forward and back. Holding on to your baby, lift at the front, then drop at the front and lift at the back. Feel your way into this movement, until it becomes an easy, smooth, full circle that extends to your shoulders and neck. Enjoy the flowing movements.

You can also 'walk your camel', doing the same movements walking forward with knees well bent. It's sexy and funny to watch. Practise walking like this during any odd moments, to loosen the hips and make more space in the pelvis for your baby.

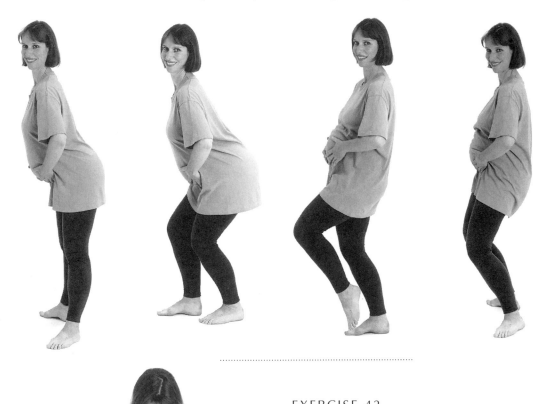

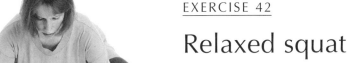

EXERCISE 42

Relaxed squat

Relax after standing and walking exercises in a deep squat. Drop your tailbone as low as it will comfortably go. Let your arms hang loose and keep the neck free and in line with the spine. The buttocks should be relaxed and the hips and pelvis wide and open.

CHAPTER 10

Floor exercises

Strengthening the birthing muscles

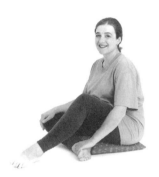

This chapter focuses on the spine, pelvis, hips and base of the body: the areas that are most affected by giving birth. All these exercises should be done as often as possible to prepare for an easy birth.

EXERCISE 43

Swan stretch

1 Kneel on the floor, on a cushion. Keep your buttocks on your heels or as near to them as possible. Spread your knees to allow room for your baby. Bring your forearms on to the floor in front of you.

2   Now stretch your arms out in front of you, as far as they will go without lifting the buttocks. This will stretch your spine, especially the lower part.

3   Push the base of your spine down on to your heels and crawl your fingers forward for maximum stretch throughout the whole trunk. Breathe easily and deeply into the extra space. This position makes more space between your ribs,

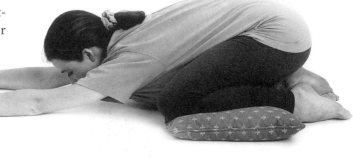

and between your ribcage and your hips, so that there is more room as your baby increases in size.

EXERCISE 44

Undulations

Having stretched throughout the length of your trunk, you are now going to move all the vertebrae in your spine in a wave-like rhythm, focusing on the back of your waist. As this part moves forward, up, back and down, all the bones that make up the spine will move too. This makes space in the spine and exercises the spinal muscles.

on the floor in front of you. Lift your buttocks off your heels and bring more weight on to your forearms. Now slide your trunk forward as far as you can without lifting your elbows from the floor.

2   When you have moved as far forward as possible, keeping your neck free and relaxed, lift your shoulders up – without moving your elbows. Feel the movement in the upper spine.

Now gently move your buttocks back towards your heels, stretching through the spine to do so. Relax your shoulders.

Repeat this circular motion several times. Breathe *in* as you come up and forward and lift your shoulders. Breathe *out* as you stretch back and down. The forearms remain on the floor all the time.

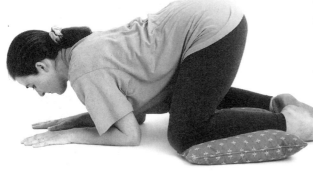

Small wave on forearms

1   Start by sitting back on your heels, with your forearms stretched out flat

Large wave on all-fours

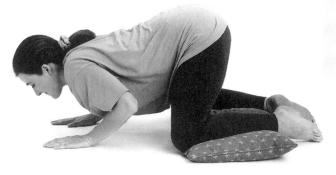

1 Sit back on your heels, as in exercise 43: Swan Stretch. Bring your weight forward on to your elbows, as before. But this time raise your elbows from the floor, so that you are taking the weight of the upper body through your wrists and on to your hands.

2 Sit back on your heels again to adjust your position. You may want to bring your elbows out a little to the sides and per-haps separate the palms more, or spread the fingers, so that your weight is evenly dis-tributed downwards from your shoulders and into your hands.

3 Lift your buttocks and bring your weight forward again, extending for-ward as far as you can. You will find that your elbows straighten, as you lift your upper back and propel it forward and up. Keep your head in line with your spine and your neck relaxed throughout.

You will feel a rhythmical rippling and undulating sensation as you exercise the different parts of your spine. As you breathe *in* you lift your buttocks, activating the lower spine. Moving through the waist, you then stretch the upper spine forward and upwards.

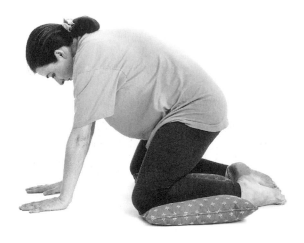

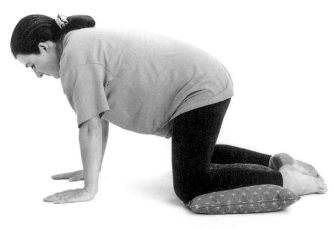

4 Move upwards and back by lifting your shoulders and 'humping' your upper back as you start to breathe *out*, getting maximum stretch in the upper back.

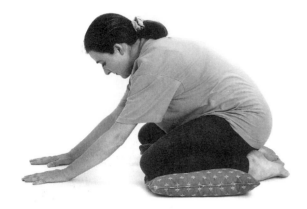

your pregnancy advances you may want to bring your heels further apart for comfort.)

6   Straighten and stretch your whole spine as you bring your forearms back on to the floor. Your waist has now completed a full circle. It is the middle back that is strong and active. The rest of the body obliges by shifting position accordingly.

5   Then start to sit back on your heels, tucking your tailbone under to get maximum stretch in your lower back. Allow your buttocks to soften and spread as wide as possible as you sit down on them. (As

Repeat this exercise several times. Do it frequently to bring flexibility and relief to your spine. It is one of the key exercises for pregnancy. Rest afterwards in exercise 43: Swan Stretch (page 85).

EXERCISE 45

Forward stretch with arm circling

If you can not reach your toes without bending your knee, you can loop a tie or belt around your instep and hold on to that. Your hips will soon get more flexible with yoga practice.

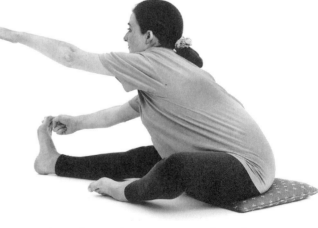

1   Sit on your cushion. Bend your left knee to the side. Keep your right leg straight with your toes turned up, so that the back of your leg is stretched throughout this exercise. Now lean forward and hold on to your right big toe with your right thumb and index finger, or hook your index and second fingers around it.

2   Breathe *in*. As you start to breathe *out*, raise your left arm and stretch it out in front of you as far as you can. This will open the base of your spine on the left side.

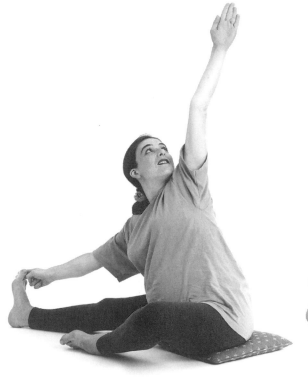

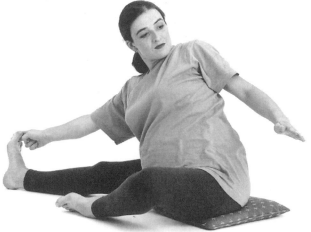

3   Start to breathe *in* again, as you sweep your straight left arm up, over and behind you, still holding your right big toe with your right hand. Follow the movement of your hand with your eyes, as you stretch all the left side of your body.

4   Breathing *out*, bring your left arm down in a sweeping circle, to start again from the beginning.

Repeat this movement, with the breathing, several times. Repeat the same number of circles with your right arm, holding on to the left foot with the left hand.

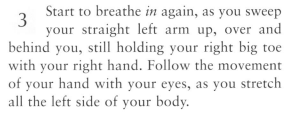

EXERCISE 46

Sitting pretty

Relax in an easy seated position, with both knees bent. One knee can drop to the side, while the other remains upright with the foot planted on the floor. Change legs frequently. This relaxed seated position helps to loosen the hip joints. You can sit in it to chat, read, watch television. Remember to sit up straight, in order to keep the chest open. Breathe evenly and deeply.

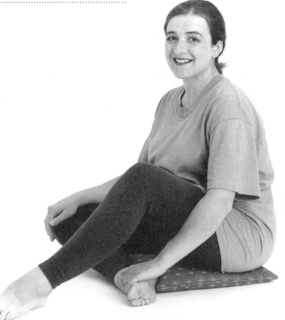

EXERCISE 47

Open position

This is one of the most useful – and simple – exercises of all. It can be done in any spare moment, so do practise it frequently between your yoga sessions as well as during them. It is a key position for good birthing as it opens the base of the body as wide as possible so that the muscles are prestretched before the birth. This ensures that they will open easily to let the baby pass through and also quickly regain their tone after the birth.

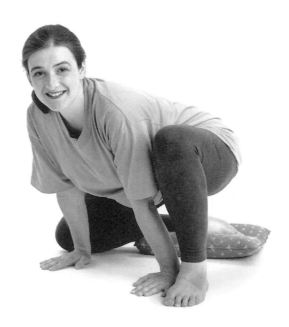

1 From exercise 46: Sitting Pretty, bring your left foot round to the side and place your hands on the floor in front of you. This will create a strong stretch across the base of the body. Raise your buttocks and bring your weight on to your hands.

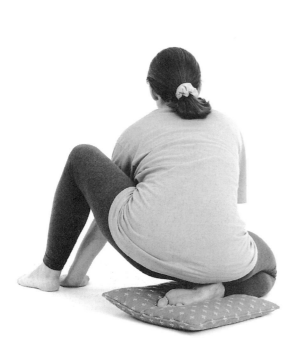

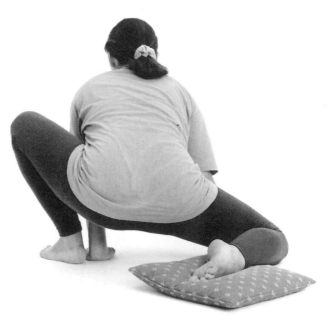

2 Shifting your front (left) foot, find the position that stretches you the most. Once you have located your most open position, stay in it for a while gently rocking back and forth for maximum stretch.

3 Practise equally on the other side, with the right foot forward.

EXERCISE 48

Knee circles

This exercise loosens the hip joints and is also very soothing. It stretches and tones the perineal muscles at the base of the body – the sooner you start practising it, the more likely you are to keep the perineum intact when your baby is born.

1 Come on to all-fours, with your knees about hips' width apart and your hands in line under your shoulders. Your spine should be stretched straight and the weight of your trunk evenly distributed through hands and knees.

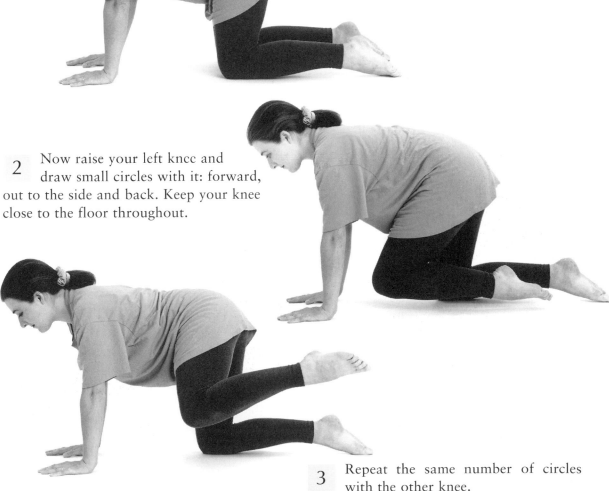

2 Now raise your left knee and draw small circles with it: forward, out to the side and back. Keep your knee close to the floor throughout.

3 Repeat the same number of circles with the other knee.

EXERCISE 49

Loose kicks and dropped hip

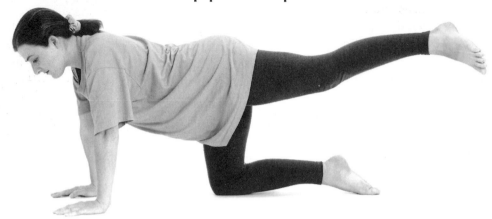

1 After doing exercise 48: Knee Circles on both sides, stretch your left knee out behind you and extend your leg loosely into a straight line parallel with the floor. Keep your head relaxed, neither dropped nor raised but in line with the spine. The aim is not to lift the straight leg, but to stretch through a horizontal line from the crown of your head to the raised foot. Avoid tension by shaking out your leg muscles in loose kicks.

2 Then lower your left leg and let it trail limply along the floor behind you. Feel your whole hip drop from the waist. Make the leg really floppy, to relax the muscles around the hips and in the thighs. Shake the whole leg in this position, as it trails behind you.

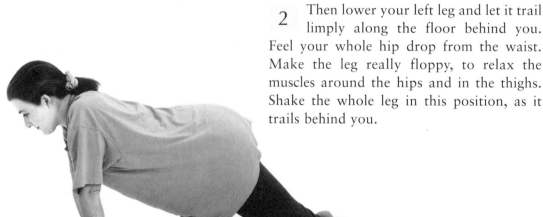

3 Come back to the all-fours position and repeat the same movements with the right leg, shaking out any stiffness or tension.

EXERCISE 50

Turtle rest

Rest with your knees wide, sitting on your heels. Bring your head to the floor, perhaps on a cushion. Tuck your chin in to lengthen the back of the neck. Bring your hands round beside your feet and relax through your shoulders. Feel your spine soft and long, and your lower back soothed.

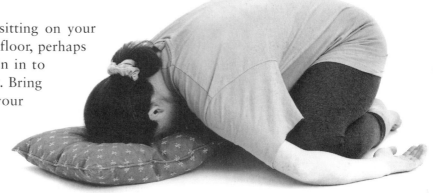

This pose is also excellent for grounding – Stage Six at the end of your deep relaxation. It marks the transition between your yoga session and the rest of the day's activities.

EXERCISE 51

Upside down

This exercise is a 'must'. Do it regularly – at first to increase your awareness of and then actively to train the groups of muscles at the base of your body that hold the baby's head in place and that will be engaged in giving birth. The more control you have over them, the fewer contractions you will need to birth your baby.

These muscles are not familiar to most women, so they can be quite hard to locate at first (see the diagram on page 121). They are easiest to find and to isolate when you are upside down, therefore start in exercise 50: Turtle Rest. Raise your buttocks off your heels, as you bring your forearms in front of you on the floor, clasping your hands. In this position, spread your elbows to the sides and bring your buttocks up, so that you are now 'upside down'. Wriggle around until you find the most comfortable position for your head and arms – so that you can forget all about them for the next few minutes.

93

1 Begin to rotate your 'tail end'. The base of the spine can move very freely in this position. Remember to breathe deeply.

2 After you have been loosening up for a while – by making small circles with the base of your spine – start to contract the muscles at the back, near the base of the spine. These are the muscles of the anus. They are strong muscles which we use automatically every time we empty our bowels. Relax and contract these muscles several times.

3 Now move your attention away from the back to the front of the base of the body. Find the muscles that you use to empty your bladder. Squeezing them may produce a tickling sensation or the urge to pass water. These muscles are inside the body, just next to the vagina.

4 Now practise squeezing up the muscles of the vagina itself, with equal pressure on the left and the right side. Then squeeze only alternate sides. It may take a while to locate and activate these muscles at will, but it is well worth persevering. It may even take several weeks to progress from dim awareness to controlled toning.

This exercise has five parts. They are:

1 Make small circles with the base of your spine (your 'tailbone').
2 Squeeze the muscles of the anus.
3 Squeeze the muscles of the bladder.
4 Squeeze the sides of the vagina.
5 Squeeze the middle of the vagina.

5 Now draw up from the *middle* of the vagina as you breathe *in*. Breathe *out* as you relax. Then breathe *in* again. Repeat this contraction and release, with the breath, several times.

Try to avoid involving the muscles of the anus or the muscles of the bladder at this stage, activating *only* the muscles of the vagina. This becomes gradually easier with practice. There is no point in over-practising.

Do this exercise about twice a week, for no more than five minutes, throughout your pregnancy to achieve the best results: awareness and control. At first the movements can quickly become tiring, but practice brings awareness and so they soon get easier. When you have done enough, stretch your legs with exercise 49: Loose Kicks and Dropped Hip (page 92). After that you may want to stand up and stretch, and shake out your legs.

WATCHPOINT

Do not hold your breath at any time during this exercise. Keep breathing deeply and evenly.

CHAPTER 11

Exercises with breath, energy and sound

Vocal power to help birthing

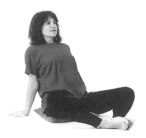

These exercises using sound can follow on from your Stage Two breathing exercises, before you get up from the floor and start moving more vigorously. Alternatively they can come at the end of your Stage Three specific routines, as you start winding down for relaxation.

Sit in a comfortable position for breathing – probably the one you have been using to centre yourself at the beginning of your yoga practice – with your spine erect, chest open and knees to the sides. Here are three examples: one is shown on the right and two overleaf.

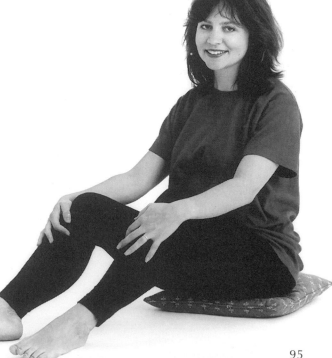

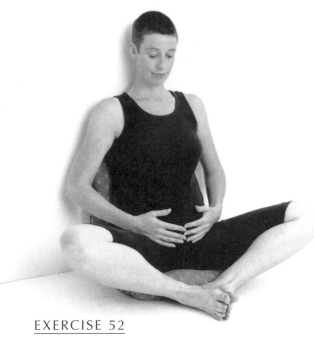

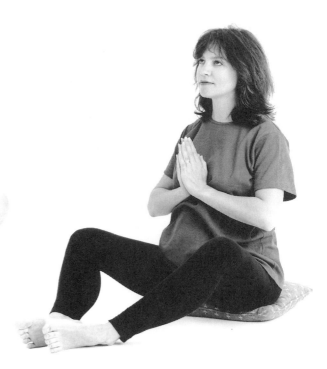

EXERCISE 52

'Aah!'

1 Breathe *in* and breathe *out*, exclaiming *'Aha!'* – as though you had just found the solution to a problem. Breathe *in* again and breathe *out*, exclaiming *'Aah...'* – as though you were sharing a friend's experience. Breathe *in* again and breathe *out*, exclaiming *'Aah...'* – as though you were taking off your shoes to relieve your tired feet after a hard day. You may even find yourself yawning deeply at this point, which is even better!

Repeat this sequence a few times, to connect with the use of sound as an expression from within. Where in your body is the expression coming from?

The first *'Aah!'* is likely to come from your head as you imagine you have just recognized or discovered something.

The second *'Aah...'* is more of an emotional response, an 'Oh dear!' coming from the energy in your heart centre as you empathize with your friend. Feel it resonating deeply in your chest.

The third *'Aah...'* is a sigh, representing a deep experience of relaxation in your body. Draw it out into a long, blissful *'Aaaah...'* It is likely to come from low down in your abdomen, and to reverberate throughout your whole body.

Practise this exercise to become familiar with the way energy expresses itself through non-verbal sounds.

2 Next, find your most effective 'note' – the best personal expression for *you* at this moment, as you are feeling now. You may need to experiment a bit, sounding a long *'Aaaah...'* several times. Breathe your sound – or sound your breath – *out* slowly and smoothly. Breathe *in* again naturally and rest a moment. Then repeat. You may find that you feel a vibration in your body right away, or that you need to try a higher or a lower note to get it, or that your voice needs to be louder, firmer or more inward, to connect with your own energies. This note is for *you*. Unlike speaking, it is not projected towards anyone else, for no one else is involved.

Experiment with your sounds, noticing which ones produce a vibration and where in your body you are feeling it. Rest after every few breaths. Remember to keep your posture aligned and upright. Let the '*Aaah...*' on your breath *out* gradually get longer and stronger.

This type of breathing is very pleasant and soothing, as the sound enhances the effect of the long breath *out*. With a little practice your '*Aaah...*' should start at the collarbones and roll down through the spine to the base of your body. The higher up in your body that the vibration starts, the higher the note is likely to be that will emerge from your mouth.

Keep your throat open and relaxed and let the sound come by itself. Feel that you are surrendering from the heart. This is actually how a baby starts being born: the baby initiates the birthing when it is ready, and the mother surrenders and allows the contractions to do all the work.

These breathing exercises, using sound, will help you to keep 'in tune' with your body's birthing process and also to help actively when you are required to do so.

EXERCISE 53

'Prrr...'

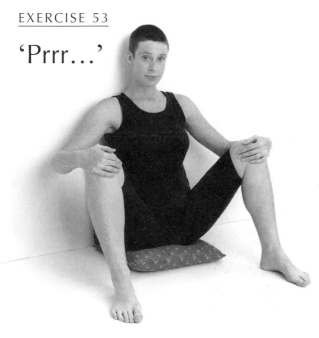

3 Now blow out '*Prrr...., Prrr....,*' very gently, rolling your Rs and purring like a happy cat. Notice the difference: there is no movement or vibration within the body.

Nothing happens because the breath is now disengaged from the spine. This knowledge gives you control over the perineum. At the time when your baby is being born you will be able to disengage your breath – together with its energy – from the strong and sometimes overwhelming contractions that bring your baby out into the world. This is an important skill. It is sometimes necessary to be able to wait for the 'birth passage' to be fully stretched and open before 'bearing down' the baby's head and shoulders through it. This '*Prrr...*' exercise can help to prevent undue haste, which may cause strain and tearing.

Then, when it is time to push, you can change your breathing pattern accordingly.

1 Sit with knees bent and feet apart, soles on the floor.

2 Lean back against the wall. Wriggle around until you find the best spot for grunting '*Huh!*' really loudly – and feeling the perineum (at the base of the body) move freely with the explosive sound.

EXERCISE 54

'Huh!'

This is the grunting breath that moves the perineum, where all the action will be when you 'bear down'. When you feel you 'want to push' – which is the phrase used by most midwives – synchronizing the contraction with breathing *out* and down the spine is a great help. Grunting *'Huh!'* activates all the muscles that will move your baby downwards. Your sound may change into a *'Haah!'* or a *'Hooh!'* on a higher or lower note. Let it! It all helps to develop your awareness of voluntary muscle action in the abdomen and perineum. You can practise 'targeting' specific muscle groups by locating the effect of your sound at various levels between the diaphragm and the base of the body.

Practise both *'Prrr...'* and *'Huh!'*, so that these exercises become second nature – to be used as appropriate without your having to think about them.

This exercise, and the following one, will prevent incontinence by strengthening the pelvic floor muscles through deep breathing. *'Huh!'* grunting is also a long-term prevention for prolapse and incontinence, which may be the outcome of over-strenuous childbirth and become an ongoing nuisance.

EXERCISE 55

'Aaaah...'

1 Breathe *out* a long *'Aaaah...'* all the way down the spine. Then draw in and quickly release the pelvic floor muscles (see the diagram on page 121). It may take a little time to become aware of these muscles that hold your 'insides' inside your body, despite the pull of gravity.

2 Breathe *in* again and repeat the exercise. Do it several more times, to get in touch with these muscles.

3 Breathe *in* again and release the breath *out* on a long *'Aaaah...'* going all the way down from top to bottom of the spine.

A few minutes at a time is enough for these breathing exercises using sound. Do, however, practise them regularly. When you are really familiar with them you can add the variations given below and practise them also.

EXERCISE 56

Cooling the soup

Birthing involves only the uterus surrounding the baby – and the breath. This is because the breath is able to activate, in a controlled way, the muscles involved in birthing. Everything else relaxes. Contractions can be 'sharp' or they can be 'deep'.

If they are 'sharp', it is best to use short, shallow breaths. Imagine blowing on hot liquid to cool it, pursing up your lips and emitting a voiceless 'Hoo' sound. Practise repeating this sound rapidly in little pants, letting the breath come *in* and go *out* by itself. Focus your attention high up – away from the abdomen, where the action is – into the upper chest and throat.

You will want to dissipate the energy of your breath, by blowing it out, only when you need to 'stop the train' of your contractions. Otherwise you will be using all of your breath, by breathing right down and involving all your abdominal muscles. They get really hard and vibrate. Deep, long breaths are best for deep, long contractions.

There are two horizontal levels of muscles in the body: the pelvic floor and the diaphragm (see the diagrams on pages 121 and 120). They are the key to giving birth, for they are the 'plungers' or 'pistons'. The downward pressure should be central and focused – much like slowly pushing down the plunger in a coffee pot. Then labour becomes smooth and easy. An experienced mother can give birth on one long breath, once the baby is in place to be pushed out.

Tension wastes energy, so you will use your yoga skills to relax from the time one contraction has peaked until the next one has arrived. You will practise long, deep breathing *out*, allowing the outside air to refill your lungs naturally, rather than 'taking' a breath *in*. In this way you can 'ride the waves'.

EXERCISE 57

'Hah...' and 'Aah!'

You can use different sounds, depending where you want to focus your energy. A sighing 'Hah...' will reach the heart space. A firm 'Aah!' will bring renewed vigour to the navel area. When you feel 'at the end of your tether' you can take your attention to your crown and roll a long 'Aaaah...' down from there, feeling it travel all the way down your spine.

Practise voicing all these sounds so that you can co-ordinate – and control – your breathing, sound and relaxation together.

CHAPTER 12

Useful labour and birthing positions

Opening the pelvis

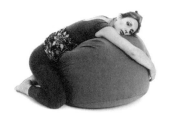

The pelvis needs to be opened to its maximum to allow the baby to pass through. Three basic positions will facilitate this opening. They are: reclining against support, squatting deeply and leaning forward. These three positions work with gravity rather than against it, allowing the baby to slip naturally downward through the birth canal (the vagina) and out into the world. Try out the various positions that follow, to find which are most comfortable and feel most 'opening'. Keep practising several alternatives that suit you, so that you can vary your position as required throughout your labour. You should change position frequently with exercise 36: Charlie Chaplin (page 77) and exercise 41: Camel Wobble (page 84) in between.

EXERCISE 58

Reclining

You can either lean back on your hands or against support. Lean back and experiment until you find the best angle. The base of the body should feel free and there should be no tension in the muscles of the lower abdomen. Check by doing the movements explained in exercise 51: Upside Down (page 93) – which require plenty of practice throughout your pregnancy, so that you are ready to use them when the time comes. You will have found a good angle when all the relevant muscles can be activated on the breath *out*. Do not wait until the birth to sort out which angle gives the best control.

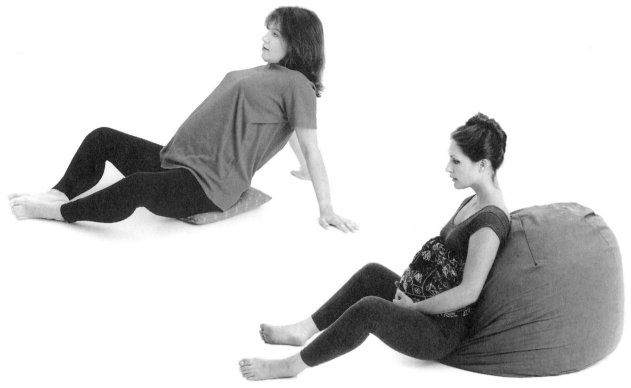

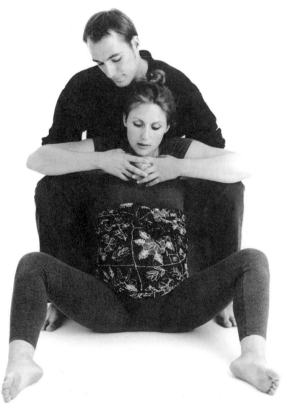

This type of position is good if you are lying on a bed during labour. The back rest on a hospital bed can be adjusted to just the right angle to lean against. Focus on mobilizing the relevant abdominal muscles, breathing *out* during the 'bearing down' contractions. Keep your legs soft and your lower jaw relaxed. There is no need to tuck your chin in, nor to make 'pushing' efforts!

The support of your partner can help you to breathe more fully. You can use your diaphragm to press down like a plunger as you breathe *out*, once your baby's head has moved down into the birth canal and is ready to appear. This is very effective and avoids straining other muscles in the body.

EXERCISE 59

Supported squatting

You can also use your diaphragm as a plunger, while breathing *out*, in a squatting position. You will need support for this. Your partner can sit on the front of a chair with knees wide and feet firmly planted on the floor, while you squat down close in front of him and between his feet.

In this position you are well supported, and so is he (by the chair and the floor). You can press down hard on his knees with your forearms. The closer your back is to his body, the more supported you will feel. Adjust both your positions, until you can feel comfortable squatting with your feet flat on the floor and your tailbone dropped down as low as possible. Find the best width between your feet and knees by working your pelvic floor muscles. (See Reclining, page 100.)

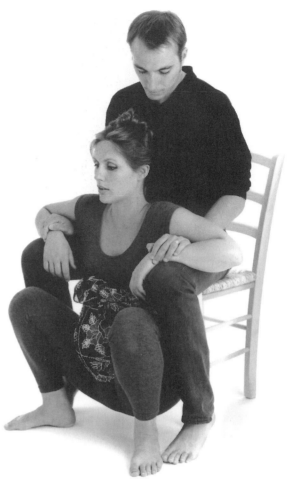

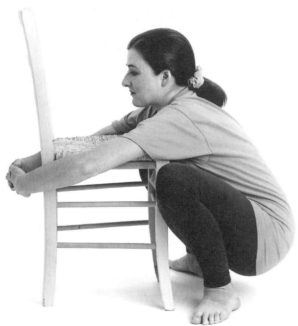

You can also squat using the support of a chair or a bed. You may feel that the base of the body is freer when you are leaning forward in a deep squat. This is a good position during the first stage of labour, while the opening from the womb is stretching. You may want to stay in it for only a few minutes at a time – unless you find squatting relaxing. This is why it is important to practise alternative positions as well.

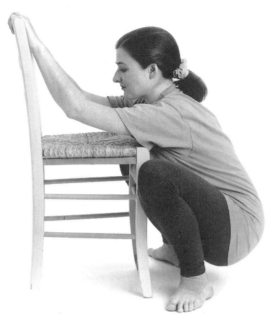

'Hanging' from a chair, with arms raised, is a good position for birthing. The breathing can be deeper, with better use of the diaphragm. You can also 'hang' from the top rail of the back rest, if you are on a hospital bed.

EXERCISE 60

Open position

(See exercise 47, page 90.) If you do not find it easy to squat deeply, this is a good alternative as it is easier to maintain for some time, with or without a chair.

Place one knee, and the opposite foot, on the floor. Move your standing foot forward and to the side until you find the most 'opening' position possible. Then bring your

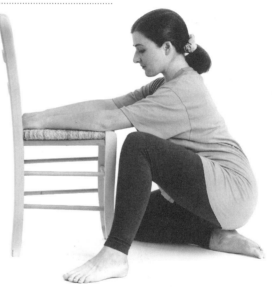

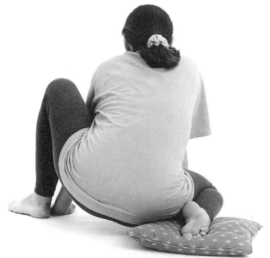

buttocks down close to the floor, so that you feel the base of your body suspended between your thighs like an old-fashioned carriage between its wheels. Now lean forward and support your weight on your arms – placing them either on the floor (or bed) in front of you or on a chair. This is often the most opening position for Western women who are not accustomed to squatting, as it allows maximum stretch at the base of the body while avoiding pressure.

EXERCISE 61

Upper back stretch

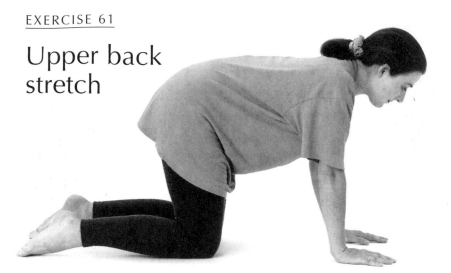

Some women find it easier to 'bear down' from the upper part of the back – which must therefore be stretched and well supported. The all-fours position is excellent for this (see exercise 48: Knee Circles, page 91).

Keeping the spine stretched in a straight line, spread out your hands to take your weight and place your knees far enough apart to allow maximum opening at the base of the body. Feel the buttocks spreading and relaxing.

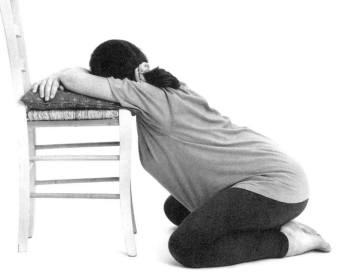

WATCHPOINT

Symmetry is important. Make sure that your hands are placed squarely beneath your shoulders and your knees are in line with your hips. This ensures alignment of the spine. Your waist should not sag at the back, nor should your head either droop or poke upwards.

The same alignment can be achieved, but with greater support, by resting your fore-arms on a chair or bed. This position helps you to synchronize your breath *out* with the birthing contractions, feeling the action happening all the way from your upper back to the base of the body. The lower back is also well stretched in this position, avoiding pressure and strain. These two positions are particularly helpful if your baby is facing forwards, or if you have already had a caesarian section.

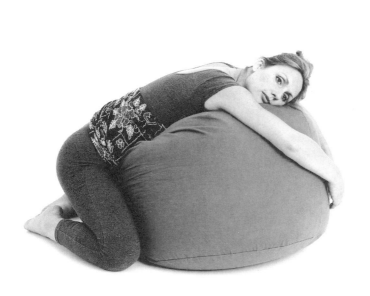

You can achieve the same symmetrical alignment and full spinal stretch, in a more relaxed manner, by draping yourself over a beanbag or pile of bolsters and blankets.

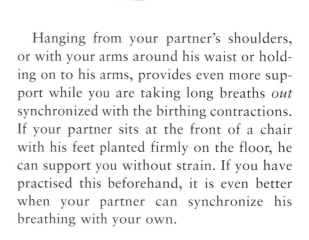

Hanging from your partner's shoulders, or with your arms around his waist or holding on to his arms, provides even more support while you are taking long breaths *out* synchronized with the birthing contractions. If your partner sits at the front of a chair with his feet planted firmly on the floor, he can support you without strain. If you have practised this beforehand, it is even better when your partner can synchronize his breathing with your own.

EXERCISE 62

Braking position

Sometimes you may need to slow down for respite, when contractions are coming fast and furiously. Sometimes a midwife advises you *not* to 'push' yet, although you are already getting the urge to 'bear down'. On such occasions you can go into the Upside Down position described on page 93.

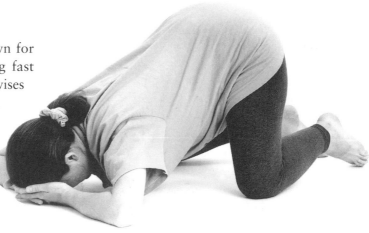

....

EXERCISE 63

Preparation with massage and breathing

In order for the base of the body to be yielding, and to stretch without tearing, it is important to prepare the tissues inside the vagina properly. One method is through massage, the other through breathing. You can either recline in the position shown in the photograph on page 101 (right) or support yourself on a chair in the position shown in the photograph on page 103 (right), but keeping one hand free.

Massage

Massage should be gentle stroking without pressure to encourage blood flow. Explore the area with a light touch. Learn to differentiate between the anal and vaginal tissues. It is the vaginal tissues which will be the most stretched. If you have had tears during

a previous birthing, focus particularly on those areas.

You can relax and help the blood circulation by having a soothing bath first, or by applying a hot flannel, or by using a light oil (such as almond).

The nipples require the same gentle attention, as you recline against support. Massage of the nipples stimulates the production of hormones involved in labour and birth, as well as preparing for breastfeeding. It is most effective when combined with deep breathing *and* pelvic floor lifts (see exercise 51: Upside Down, page 93.)

Breathing

Here you use your fingers passively, simply as a focus to breathe against. The stretching comes from within the tissues themselves, on the breath *out*.

Insert two fingers into the vagina up to the first knuckle, progressing to the second knuckle with practice. Press firmly but gently against the back wall of the vagina, towards the spine. Breathe deeply, until you can feel the involvement of the muscles under your fingers every time you breathe *out*. When you become aware of extra space, you can start exerting a little more pressure. You will be amazed how much stretching takes place with regular practice! The more you pre-stretch before the birth, the better you will return to your original shape afterwards.

Preparing your perineum for birth through use of breathing exercises can be compared to stretching a balloon. At first you may feel that nothing much is happening as you blow. Then your perineal tissue – like the rubber of the balloon – starts giving and stretches to the desired size.

These exercises can avoid tearing and are especially useful if you have had a tear or cut during a previous birth. They help with birthing 'lightly', making full use of the breath.

WATCHPOINT

Practise only five to eight minutes at a time. Keep your fingers as a lever, passive against your breathing. There should be no manual attempt to stretch mechanically.

CHAPTER 13

Completing a yoga session

Winding down, relaxation, grounding

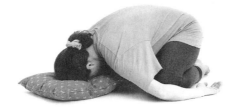

STAGE FOUR

Winding down

Prepare for relaxation before you begin your yoga session, so that you can slip into it smoothly when you have finished your exercise routines. Have extra clothing handy, as your body will cool down. Have ready extra padding, cushions, beanbag and so on, so that you can make yourself really comfortable and stay in your chosen position without moving for ten minutes or more. If you are playing yourself a relaxation tape, have it ready to switch on.

Part of your winding-down ritual is to get warm and comfortable. Take time to settle

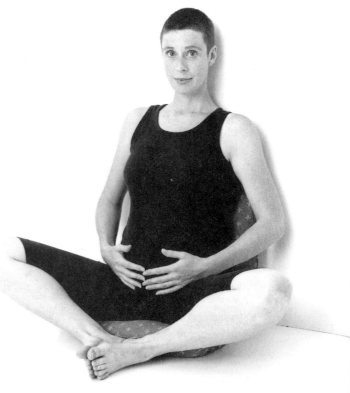

yourself in a seated position, leaning on cushions against a wall or on a beanbag.

If you are less than 30 weeks pregnant, you may prefer to lie down, either flat on your back or with your legs supported. Cushions or a beanbag can be very comfortable.

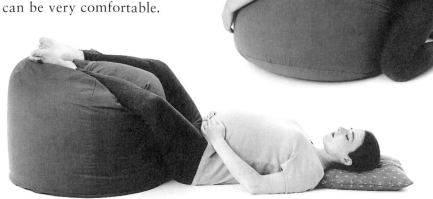

Centre yourself inwards by lying or sitting quietly and breathing deeply, with the elbows bent and palms together. This brings your energy into your personal centre – the place you feel is 'me'. Slow breathing will slow the rate of the heartbeats. This, in turn, will relax the mind. If you are sitting up, this is a good time to practise some of the sound exercises in Chapter 11 to take your focus inwards.

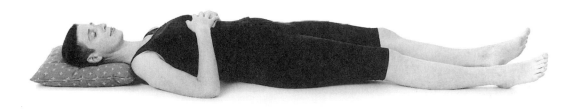

STAGE FIVE

Deep relaxation

Deep relaxation is about being in the moment, being aware of the sensations and feelings that arise from within, accepting whatever comes – and then letting go, without thought or comment, of all that we no longer feel we want to keep.

We accumulate a lot of emotional 'clutter' simply through the process of living.

Relaxation can be a sorting process, at a very deep level. It can be an opportunity to choose and cherish whatever supports us and gives joy – whatever helps us to feel more in tune with life itself, and more loving towards those who are sharing life with us.

Relaxation can also be an opportunity to clear away old habits of fear and insecurity;

to let go of past hurts and all that limits our ability to grow into our potential for love and joy. This choice is made from the heart, rather than the mind. In relaxation we simply witness what arises – and release it if it no longer serves us.

It is a good idea to reflect upon the above explanation of deep relaxation, so that you are open to the long-term emotional well-being that it can bring, as well as the physical benefits.

Entering the relaxed state

To enter a deeply relaxed state you can focus your mind for a while on the gentle rhythm of your breath. You may want to scan your body mentally for residual tension: check your neck, shoulders, spine, abdomen, arms, legs, small joints. Breathe *out* into any parts that are holding tension – let it float away with the breath.

Alternatively you can place your hands around your baby to create a circle of love enclosing both of you, and breathe *in* and *out* of your heart centre. It all depends how you feel – now, for this particular relaxation session. You may feel that your heart is open and relaxed, in touch with your baby. If so, just breathe into your heart space and keep this connection going. There is a joint dynamic between mother and baby. The more you can keep your focus in the heart during relaxation, the easier it is to maintain this precious link during the birth.

You may prefer instead to play a relaxation tape that you have recorded and just follow the words to take you deeper. Below are two relaxations, of different lengths and content, for you to put on tape and play back to yourself. Make your voice serene and happy as you read them slowly, with frequent pauses, so that your mind can pick up the words without any effort or disturbance of its tranquillity. You may like your partner to read one or both of them, if this gives you pleasure and a feeling of shared experience. Experiment with making your relaxation tapes, until you are happy with the results. Switch on when you feel settled and your body has let go of tensions.

First relaxation: five minutes

This can be practised by couples on a regular basis, at the end of the breathing sessions they do together. It works best when the breathing of the two prospective parents is synchronized. This happens naturally with practice and can be a wonderful experience.

Record the words from here and play the tape back during your relaxation as soon as you are settled and comfortable:

Breathe *out* deeply a couple of times, focusing your awareness on the base of your spine. Whether you are lying down or sitting up, start easing out your lower back. Feel that your pelvis is sinking down, as though into warm sand. Feel your buttocks softening and spreading out.

Find what seems to you to be the centre of your body. Breathe *in* to this area. As you breathe *out*, become aware of your arms and legs. Breathe *in* again. Next time you breathe *out*, let your arms and legs relax all at once. Let them flop completely on the breath *out*. Breathe *in* again and flop even more as you breathe *out*. Really let go...

Feel how relaxed your arms and shoulders are now... Bring your attention to your neck. Move your head a little. Align it with your spine, so that your neck feels free and comfortable... Drop your lower jaw and relax all the muscles around your mouth.

Are your eyes softly closed? If not, close them now. Take your attention inwards. Feel interested in, and receptive to, whatever you may find there. Welcome yourself, just as you are now. Let yourself simply *be*... Acknowledge and welcome whatever may arise from within your deeper self – whether thoughts, emotions or images. Accept them, just as they are.

Now focus on your heart area. A great expansion of feeling is taking place here, preparing for your baby, just as your womb is expanding to allow your baby to grow within it. Feel the space that you are creating in your heart – and in your life, as well as in your body – to welcome this new person.

Allow yourself to connect with the wonder of this expanding new space. Feel how it also enriches you and all your loved ones. Feel how it spreads its warmth to everyone around you. Trust that you have all the resources you need, both within yourself and from outside yourself, to be the happy mother of a happy child.

Silently convey this assurance to your unborn child, again and again...

Become aware once more of your breathing, as it flows *in* and *out*. Start to bring yourself back to outer awareness and activity. Gradually expand your breathing, until you feel your eyes ready to open by themselves. Let them open and gaze around you, slowly letting the world around you come into focus...

When you are ready, start to move gently. Come on to all-fours. Rock yourself back and forth for a moment or two. Then ground yourself before getting up.

Second relaxation: fifteen minutes, with music and visualization

For this relaxation, record the following words to begin your tape:

Once you are comfortably settled for deep relaxation, start to focus your awareness on your lower back. Be aware of the base of your spine. This becomes a door through which you can enter a deeper and deeper state of relaxation. You can access this state during your pregnancy, during your labour and also after your baby has been born.

Breathe *in* and then breathe *out*, as deeply as you can, down your spine and into your lower back. You may like to do this again, voicing an 'Aaah...' sound. Sometimes this sound may help you to release unsuspected tension as you breathe *out*. Notice if it has this effect...

Let your relaxation spread out from your lower back. Feel it spreading downwards into your buttock muscles, thigh muscles, calves... Feel it spreading upwards all through the muscles of your back, so that they spread out and soften... Let the muscles of your shoulders and arms relax – all the way from the inner back to the palms of your hands... Feel how floppy your arms and legs have become, and how the soles of your feet and the palms of your hands are now open and soft.

Bring your awareness to the area around your navel, which is opposite your 'door to relaxation' in your lower back. Expand your breathing in this navel area. This is second nature to you by now. You are accustomed to breathing deeply into your navel area. Your baby has also grown used to your expanded breathing at the navel. Your rhythms are now familiar to your baby, in its fluid sac, sheltered within your womb, securely positioned in the strong, bony case of your pelvis. Enjoy your expanded breathing together.

Be receptive to any thoughts that may come to you. Welcome any sensations, feelings, emotions, that you may experience about your pregnancy and your growing baby. Let your body-mind grow quieter and quieter. Slip into neutral gear as you relax deeper and deeper. Disengage your mind, as well as your body, from all conscious activity...

Just 'be here now', very quietly, while the most astonishing growth and development is taking place within you. Experience this growth directly, more powerful than any picture or image can be. Allow all aspects of your experience to come together in their own way. Some will integrate below consciousness. Some may come to the surface and, perhaps, surprise you. Whatever your natural response, simply acknowledge your experience without identifying with it. Release whatever emotions may arise in you as a result of your experience at this time...

Notice how the whole front of your body is involved in this receptive registering of your inner feelings and sensations... Connect with your heart, to expand further your capacity to give and receive love and compassion... Feel open, trusting, ready for new experiences – of the birth, the future, the unknown... Feel receptive to change. Respond to any fears that may surface with a little message of love and trust from you to your baby, and from you to yourself as a woman... Know

that by doing this, in deep relaxation, you are consolidating the base of gentle power that is yours to rely upon – during your baby's birth and afterwards, for the rest of your life...

Connect now with your throat. Check that your lower jaw is loose, and that all the muscles around your mouth are soft and relaxed. Check that your neck is free and relaxed. Feel that your eyes are closed, soft behind your eyelids.

Start to focus on your sense of hearing, letting your other senses fade away as you withdraw them inwards into deeper relaxation. Notice any sounds outside, or around you. Let them float through you, without any need to respond to them in any way. In a moment you will hear the music that you have recorded... When it starts, take a deep breath. As you let it go, relax your whole body all at once, from the crown of your head to the soles of your feet...

Most mammals require a feeling of security when they have babies. Human beings feel the same. In fact, this is probably the most crucial feeling in the quality of the birth experience. Relaxation combined with visualization can help to develop a greater inner sense of strength, peace and security around the whole process of giving birth.

At this stage you may wish to record some relaxing music of your choice. Select a short piece of music that evokes these feelings, to match the words you will be hearing immediately afterwards. With repetition, the music will take you straight 'there', without the need for words. Natural sounds (ocean, birds, rain), with or without musical accompaniment, can be very relaxing. Trust your intuition, as you choose the particular music or recording for this pregnancy. Babies respond to sound from the fourth month of pregnancy. The voice starts again as the music fades.

You may prefer, instead of music, to have four minutes of silence in which to nurture your being – perhaps to heal past traumas – and integrate your experience. It is best to provide your own sound marker at the beginning and end of the four minutes' silence, before the voice starts again:

As the music fades away, you are left with the feeling of being totally safe, loved and in harmony with your surroundings. Picture these surroundings, conjuring up an image of a place which you know, or which you can enjoy building up in your imagination.

Use all your senses to bring this place into focus, to make it as real and solid as possible, so that you feel yourself actually there. Register the light, the colours, the textures, the temperature... Notice the feelings and associations which may come into your awareness. Are you alone, or are other people with you in this special place? Register the qualities of your feelings, especially those which enhance your sense of wellbeing and harmony, as you experience yourself in this place...

There is a way in and out of this place. Find the doorway. It may be wide or narrow, hidden or easy to see. When you have found it, pass through it – and find yourself back in the room where you are in deep relaxation.

You can return easily to your special place, and the feelings of peace and safety that it gives you... Just take a breath – and let it go, as you relax from the crown

of your head to the soles of your feet all on the one breath *out*... There you are, back in your special place! Again, find the way out and pass through it, coming back into this room where you are in deep relaxation. Practise letting go all on the one breath *out* – and finding yourself back in your special place. Then pass through the door and back into this room. Repeat this a few times...

At this point allow about two minutes' silence, while you repeat going in and out of your special place. Then it is time to come out of deep relaxation, so let the tape lead you out:

Now become aware of your breath and expand it gradually and steadily until you find that you are practising full, deep, abdominal breathing focused on your navel. You will find that your eyes want to open by themselves. Let them open and slowly focus on your surroundings. When you have returned to full body awareness, move gently into your 'grounding' position, before you stretch and get up.

If you are already in bed, you will now go to sleep. If you fell asleep during your relaxation, that is all right too. You probably needed this sleep and it has been beneficial for you. Take it as an indication that you may need more sleep than you are getting and arrange your life to allow for extra resting time. This applies especially in early and late pregnancy.

This visualization can be a great help when you are in labour. Once you have practised it regularly, it is easy to go in and out of your 'special place' and even to stay in it as you rest between contractions. Even if you do not make use of the visualization during labour, its effects will be with you. The quality of your experience during deep relaxation while pregnant creates feelings of safety and harmony that will help you to meet the challenges of labour and birth.

Once you know how to visualize, it may be helpful to store up images of beauty that you come across, so that they are available to recapture during labour. Smells are always powerfully evocative, as are tunes you learn to sing or chant. Practise recapturing happy experiences in your mini relaxations.

STAGE SIX

Grounding

It is important to have practised what you do *after* relaxation before you begin!

As the sounds on the tape die away, prepare to return to everyday awareness. Take it slowly. Come out of your relaxation position by bending the elbow and knee on the same side, and rolling over to that side and then on to all-fours.

Finally, 'ground' yourself before getting up. Always use a simple ritual to mark the transition between your yoga session and the next thing on your agenda. Placing your hands on the floor, and perhaps your head as well, is grounding.

Taking stock of how you feel now, after your yoga session, is also grounding. So is tidying up your yoga space, or eating and drinking.

If you rush straight out through the door without grounding yourself, you may lose the peacefulness that you have been building up. The deeper your relaxation, the more important it is to come out of it slowly and completely before starting on something else. However long or short your yoga session has been, do make sure that you always start with Stage One: Centring and finish with Stage Six: Grounding.

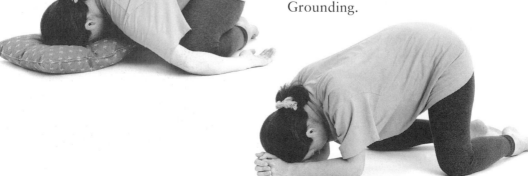

CHAPTER 14

Beanbag sequence

An exercise session

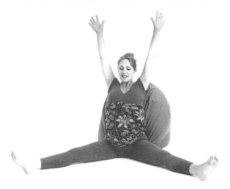

This chapter outlines a balanced, short programme suitable for late pregnancy. A good, full beanbag is a most useful accessory as it allows you to work to a rhythm of stretching and relaxing without having to change your position, which can become laborious and tiring during the later stages of pregnancy. It can also be comforting during labour and useful after your baby is born, so it is a long-term investment.

How to use the beanbag

Lean against your beanbag, rather than sitting on top of it, to get the best support. First shake it until you can get hold of a part of the cover that is empty of beans, like an empty envelope. Smooth this flat part out on the floor and then sit on it,

so that your beanbag is firmly anchored underneath you. You can now lean comfortably against the full part behind you. If your beanbag sags a bit, place it against a wall for better support.

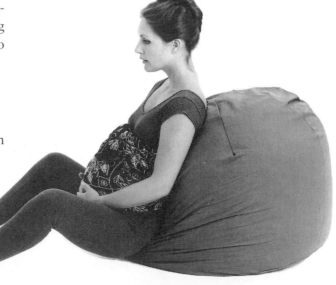

moments in this position, letting your mind and body settle. You will probably feel your baby settling as well, getting used to the quietening rhythm of your breath. Keep your neck relaxed, the shoulders loose and down. Feel that your spine is lengthening.

EXERCISE 64

Breathing

1 Settle yourself against your beanbag. Sit with knees bent and feet wide apart on the floor. Let your knees fall outwards to open the pelvic area. Place your hands around your baby. Spend a few

2 When you are ready, start to breathe slowly and deeply. As you breathe *out*, feel that you are breathing *down* the spine to the floor, right through the strong muscles at the base of the body. As you breathe *in*, feel that the breath rises *up* in the spine. This familiar breathing pattern opens the chest and makes more room for your baby on the breath *in*, and relaxes and softens the base of the body on the breath *out*.

EXERCISE 65

Forward and up

1 (This is the same as exercise 24: Peekaboo!, page 61.) Take your legs to the side as wide as you comfortably can. Let them relax, knees loose and flat against the floor. You may be surprised how supple you become when you are pregnant – it is nature's way of enabling you to adjust to the process of carrying and giving birth to a baby. Turn your toes up towards the ceiling to stretch your legs more. Keep your legs and feet in this position, while you move your trunk and arms. Bring your bent arms up, clasping opposite forearms loosely.

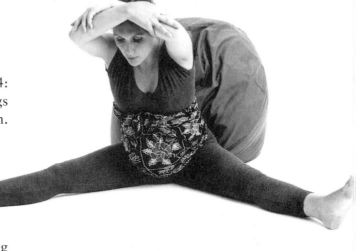

2 This immediately opens the sides of the body. As you breathe *in*, stretch your folded arms forward from the elbows to open the upper back, then up overhead to open the front of the body. Breathe *out*, as you release your clasp and float your arms gently down to the sides. Repeat several times to get a good forward and upward stretch of the upper body. Then rest with your hands clasped around your baby, before starting the next stretch. You may like to bend your knees a little as well.

EXERCISE 66

'Hooray!' stretch

1 As you breathe *in*, bring your hands up to the sides and *stretch* them up overhead. Spread your fingers and reach for the sky. Feel the energy of your breath reach right into your fingertips.

2 When you need to breathe *out*, let the arms float down again to your lap. The energy of your breath spreads down the spine to the base, and all around your baby. Your deep breathing is always a treat for your baby. Repeat this sweeping movement a few times, then rest as before. Feel your baby within the circle of your embrace.

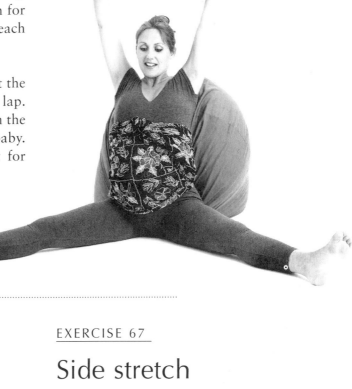

EXERCISE 67

Side stretch

1 The next movement is a side bend. As you breathe *in*, take your left arm overhead. Stretch up as high as you can, letting your right hand lie relaxed along your right leg with the palm upwards.

2 As you breathe *out*, lean to the right. Maintain the stretch all along your left side and left arm, as you lean on your right elbow. If it is comfortable for you, turn your head to look up at your left hand. If you prefer, continue to look straight ahead.

117

3   When you are ready to breathe *in* again, stretch up, bringing the spine back to centre. As you breathe *out*, lower your left arm.

4   As you breathe *in* again, raise your right arm and repeat the whole movement, leaning to the left.

Repeat this whole sequence a few times, then rest with your hands around your baby.

EXERCISE 68

Relaxation

You may wish to relax with your knees bent and rolling out to the side, as for your deep breathing exercise.

Alternatively you may prefer to place your beanbag in front of you and relax across it. Kneel with your knees wide apart and toes touching. Drape your trunk and arms across the beanbag so that it takes your weight and adjusts to your contours. This is a very soothing position, especially during the last weeks of pregnancy. It is also soothing during labour, and a position in which you can give birth.

After relaxation take several moments to come to everyday awareness before getting to your feet.

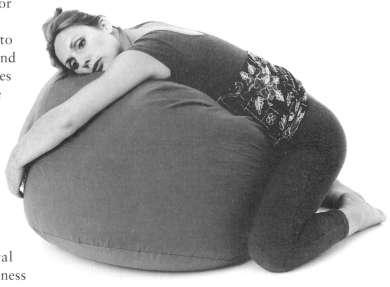

Postscript

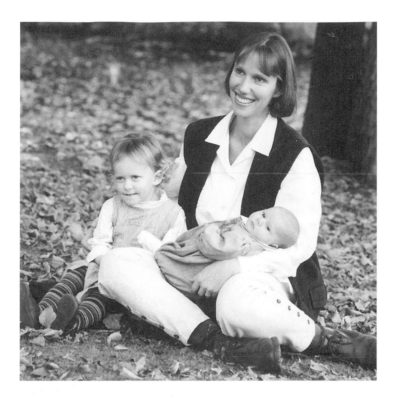

I brought Alice to the surface of the pool in the early hours of a September morning. It had been a very peaceful labour, due I'm sure to the heightened awareness our bodies and minds are able to acquire through yoga. For me, it was also particularly special to be at home and to be supported by such a sensitive midwife.

At 11pm the previous evening we walked down the lane with our two-year-old daughter, and once she had been tucked up in bed we busied ourselves topping up the pool and getting the room ready. I didn't have to recall consciously any of the excercises so useful for pain relief during the first stage – I found that my body just fell into a routine and rhythm of its own that felt right for the moment. Once I was supported by the water, all my awareness naturally centred on my breathing – yes, the contractions were painful, but they could be endured entirely by regulating my breathing. Witnessing the birth of our little one as she was literally breathed out into her new world was an experience I shall never forget.

How very fitting that Françoise should be Alice's first visitor – appearing out of the night to sit and talk softly in the candlelight – we shall always cherish that special moment along with all her care and support to us as a family.

Alison Gilderdale

Appendix

Breathing

Breathing goes on automatically all through our life. However, we can develop awareness and control of our breathing through yoga practice. We can breathe more slowly and deeply, which allows more oxygen to circulate in the bloodstream.

The chief breathing muscle is the diaphragm, separating the chest from the abdomen. Above the diaphragm are the lungs (and heart), below it are the digestive organs (and your baby). The diaphragm contracts *downwards*, synchronizing with other muscles that contract to lift the breastbone and ribs *outwards*.

As the 'breathing muscles' contract, the space in the lungs is made bigger. This causes air from outside to be drawn in, via the nose and windpipe. We call this *'breathing in'* (see diagram A).

As the 'breathing muscles' relax, the space in the lungs cavity is made smaller. This causes air to be pushed out, via the nose and windpipe. We call this *'breathing out'* (see diagram B).

Key to diagrams
1 = **Spine**
2 = **Breastbone**
3 = **Ribs** joined to spine and breastbone
4 = **Diaphragm muscle**
5 = **Lungs** (and heart) space
6 = **Abdomen**

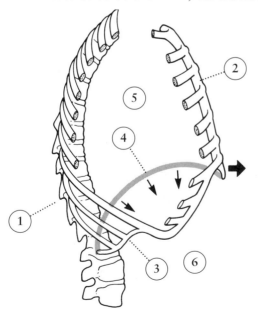

A Breathing in

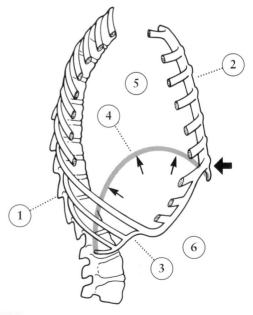

B Breathing out

The pelvic ligaments and openings in the pelvic floor

Your baby grows in your womb, which lies in your lower abdomen. The supporting muscles and ligaments – shown in a grey tint in diagrams C (five months pregnant) and D (nine months pregnant) – need to be kept well toned as the size and weight of the womb increase. This crowds the abdominal space and puts pressure on the pelvic floor (the perineum) at the base of the body.

The womb opens into the vagina, which will become the birth canal. The vagina, the openings to your large bowel, and also your bladder, all pass through the pelvic floor. The exercises in this book build up strength, awareness and control in specific muscle groups situated in the pelvic floor area.

This allows you to relax or contract these muscles, as required, and this will assist the process of birth.

Key to diagrams

1 = **Anus** (bowel opening)
2 = **Bladder opening**
3 = **Vagina** (birth canal)
(1–3 are the three openings in the pelvic floor at the base of the body)
4 = **Spine**
5 = **Pubic bone**
6 = **Large bowel**
7 = **Bladder**
8 = **Baby in womb**

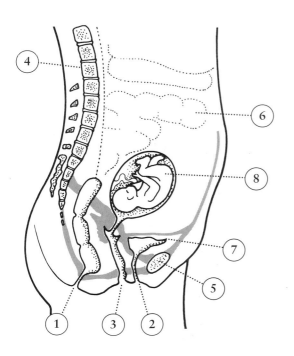

C 5 months pregnant

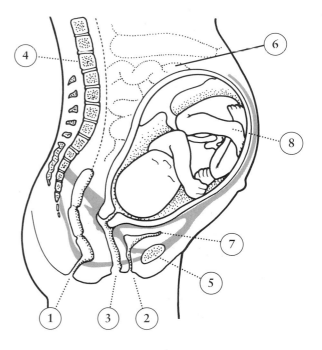

D 9 months pregnant

Troubleshooting

Yoga helps to prevent or remove many common discomforts experienced during pregnancy. However, yoga should *not* be seen as a substitute for other aspects of antenatal care. Your blood pressure should be checked at regular intervals. You should also ensure that you receive the best possible nutrition, with vitamin and mineral supplements as needed.

Most symptoms that develop during pregnancy are just part of the process. Yoga is a safe and gentle 'toolkit' that can restore and improve your wellbeing and that of your baby. Some general guidelines follow.

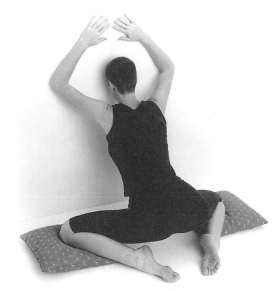

WATCHPOINT

If you experience severe pain or bleeding, stop whatever you are doing – including your yoga practice – and seek medical help right away.

Aches in the groin

These are due to the extra pressure and stretching. The remedy is to practise standing squats and the exercises in Chapter 7 to loosen up around the hips and pelvic floor.

Anxiety and stress

After a hard day, for whatever reason, turn for help to your yoga. Deep relaxation with visualization will calm fears, deep breathing/energy work will restore harmony and peace, energetic routines will bring back your sense of wellbeing and joy.

Heartburn

Sit in a posture that makes more space below the diaphragm, so that the digestive process is not cramped. Keep the spine erect, using cushions or a wall. Keep your breastbone lifted up throughout your deep breathing/energy practice – even while breathing *out* slowly. Raise and lower your arms to open the sides of the body more. See Chapter 6. Up to 36 weeks only: kneel in front of a wall and press your hands hard against it, pressing your shoulderblades together to open the front of the body more.

Muscle cramps

Standing and all-fours routines help the circulation. So do deep breathing and relaxation (up to 30 weeks, with legs up the wall). Cramps are caused by lack of oxygen in the muscle. Other remedies are: sipping water slowly, massage and pressing the points on the inside of the ankle or between the big and second toes.

Non-specific lower backache

Up to 30 weeks, resting your legs up the wall is a great help. Throughout your pregnancy the exercises in Chapters 9 and 10 will improve energy flow and muscle tone in this area.

Piles and varicose veins

Practise exercise 51: Upside Down (page 93) frequently, both for relief of piles and for muscle toning to prevent them. Up to 30 weeks, exercise 5: Legs up the Wall (page 43) is generally helpful. The wide-legged positions in Chapter 6 and seated deep breathing/energy practice with soles touching are useful throughout pregnancy to relieve varicose veins in the legs. Rotate your ankles gently at odd moments.

Sciatic pain

The all-fours exercises in Chapter 10 are a 'must'! Be gentle but persistent with the side that hurts. Dropping the hip and small knee circles reduce stiffness when you get up and lessen pain at the end of the day.

Sleeplessness and exhaustion

Deep relaxation and energy breathing help to restore vitality when you feel tired. The energetic routines help to provide a reservoir of vitality for you to draw upon, so that you do not get tired so easily. Use your own judgement – do you need rest or exercise right now? You *always* need energy breathing! It also helps you to sleep well.

Swollen joints

Again, improving the circulation is a great help. Practise the energetic routines in Chapters 6 and 9. Drink plenty of water. Gently rotate the ankle and wrist joints in spare moments.

Uncomfortably 'heavy' breasts

Sitting with the breastbone lifted improves muscle tone. So does pressing the palms together at heart level. See Chapter 6.

List of addresses

The following addresses are sources of further information:

Active Birth Centre
55, Dartmouth Park Road
London NW5 1SL
Tel: 0171 267 3006
Fax: 0171 267 5368

Association of Radical Midwives
62, Greetby Hill
Omskirk
Lancashire L39 2DT

Birthlight
Stable House
19 High Street
Little Shelford
Cambridge CB2 5ES
Tel: 01223 845 508
Fax: 01223 845 509

British Wheel of Yoga
Central Office
1, Hamilton Place
Boston Road
Sleaford, Lincs.
NG34 7ES
Tel: 01529 306 851

Home Birth Movement
10, Portrush Close
Woodley
Reading, Berkshire
RG5 9PB

La Leche League International
(Great Britain)
Box 3424
London WC1N 3XX
Tel: 0171 242 1278

Maternity Alliance
45, Beach Street
London EC2P 2LX
Tel: 0171 588 8582

National Childbirth Trust
Alexandra House
Oldham Terrace
Acton
London W3 6NH
Tel: 0181 922 8637

National Health Information Service
Freephone 0800 665 544

Ruth White Yoga Centre
Church Farm House
Springclose Lane
Cheam
Surrey SN3 8PU
Tel/Fax: 0181 644 0309

Satyananda Yoga Centre
70, Thurleigh Road
Balham
London SW12 8UD
Tel: 0181 673 4869

USA
International Childbirth Education
Association (ICEA)
PO Boc 20048
Minneapolis
MN 55 420

Birth Resources
1749, Vine Street
Berkeley
CA 94703

List of exercises in this book

Index

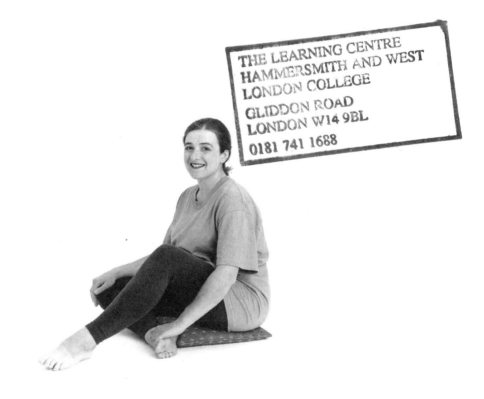